Confessions
of a Surgeon

Confessions of a Surgeon

The Good, the Bad, and the Complicated . . .
Life Behind the O.R. Doors

PAUL A. RUGGIERI, M.D.

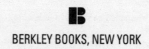

BERKLEY BOOKS, NEW YORK

THE BERKLEY PUBLISHING GROUP
Published by the Penguin Group
Penguin Group (USA) Inc.
375 Hudson Street, New York, New York 10014, USA
Penguin Group (Canada), 90 Eglinton Avenue East, Suite 700, Toronto, Ontario M4P 2Y3, Canada
(a division of Pearson Penguin Canada Inc.)
Penguin Books Ltd., 80 Strand, London WC2R 0RL, England
Penguin Group Ireland, 25 St. Stephen's Green, Dublin 2, Ireland (a division of Penguin Books Ltd.)
Penguin Group (Australia), 250 Camberwell Road, Camberwell, Victoria 3124, Australia
(a division of Pearson Australia Group Pty. Ltd.)
Penguin Books India Pvt. Ltd., 11 Community Centre, Panchsheel Park, New Delhi—110 017, India
Penguin Group (NZ), 67 Apollo Drive, Rosedale, Auckland 0632, New Zealand
(a division of Pearson New Zealand Ltd.)
Penguin Books (South Africa) (Pty.) Ltd., 24 Sturdee Avenue, Rosebank, Johannesburg 2196,
South Africa

Penguin Books Ltd., Registered Offices: 80 Strand, London WC2R 0RL, England

This is an original publication of The Berkley Publishing Group.

PRINTING HISTORY
Berkley trade paperback edition / January 2012

Library of Congress Cataloging-in-Publication Data

Ruggieri, Paul, 1959–
    Confessions of a surgeon : the good, the bad, and the complicated—: life behind the O.R. doors /
Paul A. Ruggieri.—1st ed.
      p. cm.
    ISBN 978-0-425-24515-6
    1. Ruggieri, Paul, 1959–   2. Surgeons—Biography.   I. Title.
    RD27.35.R84 2012
    617.092—dc23
    [B]

                                                                                    2011038205

PRINTED IN THE UNITED STATES OF AMERICA

10   9   8   7   6   5   4   3   2   1

The publisher does not have any control over and does not assume any responsibility for author or
third-party websites or their content.

The events described in this book are the real experiences of real people. However, the author has
altered their identities and, in some instances, created composite characters. Any resemblance between
a character in this book and a real person therefore is entirely accidental.

Penguin is committed to publishing works of quality and integrity.
In that spirit, we are proud to offer this book to our readers;
however, the story, the experiences, and the words
are the author's alone.

To my father, John,
the most honest man I have ever known

Acknowledgments

I would like to thank all the patients whom I have had the privilege of knowing throughout my career. Every day I continue to be humbled by the trust and confidence they bestow on me. My patients have taught me invaluable lessons about life and have contributed to the making of a surgeon more so than they will ever know.

I would like to thank my agent, Donald Fehr, of Trident Media Group. Don's keen interest early on in this project was inspiring to me as a first-time author and his continued guidance was invaluable.

I am eternally grateful for the friendship and professional talents of Martha Murphy. Her enthusiasm and input into this project were instrumental to its success.

I am also indebted to my editor, Natalee Rosenstein, who believed in me, and all the people at the Berkley Publishing Group for their support in seeing this project to the end.

I would also like to deeply thank my parents, John (to whom this book is dedicated) and Irene. Their undying love and support have fostered my ability to view life's successes and failures with humble eyes, never forgetting the roots of my soul.

Acknowledgments

Most important, I have been blessed with members of my own family. They have been with me from the first to the last written word. I wish to thank my beautiful wife, Erin, for allowing me into her life and fueling my desire to follow a dream. Her honest and critical eye was instrumental in helping me tell my story. I would also like to thank my stepsons, Matt, Ryan, and Jack, along with our golden retriever, Chase, for their innocence and honesty. Their presence continues to keep me grounded every single day.

Contents

There are times, as you know, when if you leave someone alone he might live a year or two; while if you go in you might kill him. And the decision is often . . . not quite, but almost . . . arbitrary. But the odds are acceptable, provided you think the right thoughts. Or don't think at all, which I managed to do till then.

—Walter, a general surgeon, in Arthur Miller's *The Price*

Introduction

When I meet someone for the first time in a social setting and reveal (sooner or later) that I'm a surgeon, the reaction is often something close to awe (at least among those who don't spend their days in the world of healthcare). This unearned respect can be flattering, but the truth of the matter is I'd rather have my new acquaintance realize that I'm a human being, that I'm not perfect, that I'm not a demigod, and that surgery (as well as the rest of medicine) is an art as much as a science. And some days, calling it an art is a stretch.

Becoming a surgeon was the most difficult thing I've ever done. The training is designed to test your mental and physical endurance as much as your intelligence or skill with a scalpel. Those without a deep reservoir of desire and drive need not apply.

Yet—once through the fire, the years and years of school and residency—working as a surgeon has provided the most exhilarating times of my life. I wouldn't trade it for anything. Most days, that is . . .

On the good days, I delight in being a member of a unique club of extraordinarily talented, complex, brilliant, driven, and compassionate professionals. We're saving lives. On the bad days, I realize I'm part of a world inhabited by flawed, greedy, egotistical, and insecure practitioners (and I include myself in that description). We're making mistakes but (usually) correcting them before lasting damage is done. The middle ground looks like this: I get to work with a motley crew of healthcare professionals, surrounded by diseased organs, blood, pus, and guts, in a room without windows hidden behind a set of swinging doors, where we spend too much time on our feet but get to improve the quality of someone's life or (maybe) extend someone's life. At the end of the day, it usually feels pretty good.

My profession is complex and complicated. It demands a dedication to a way of life that is like no other. For me, the road leading into the operating room is a lonely one, the path to a place where I am responsible for all that transpires, be it good, bad, or complicated. Most days in the O.R. *do* go well (thankfully), whether the crew and I experience exhilaration, fear, boredom, satisfaction, or humiliation before we call it quits.

I love being a surgeon. I love being able to make a clear, tangible difference in the quality of a person's life. Sometimes I even save a life. I am honored every time a patient comes to me, and I'm humbled at the trust that's given. *Confessions of a Surgeon* is my love letter to all of them, but it's more than that, too. What you have in your hands is the result of my desire to share an honest, open look at this startling profession, an occupation so unfamiliar to most it may as well be taking place on the moon.

More than thirty million people a year in this country enter hospitals to undergo surgery, for conditions including bad joints, clogged heart arteries, and diseased gallbladders. Once you are wheeled into an operating room, a host of factors—the most important of which is your surgeon—come together to influence the condition in which you will leave that room. I've long wanted to push open the O.R. doors and show the public the mysterious place where lives are improved, saved, damaged, and, sometimes, lost. I wrote this book to take you right up to the operating room table and give you an up-close view of what I see as a surgeon. I want you to meet the person behind the surgical mask.

I also want you to get a glimpse of the array of demands and constraints and desires that tug at working surgeons today: A patient's conflicting family members, each with a different idea of how a loved one's condition should be addressed. Repugnant criminals whose lives you are charged with saving. Lawsuits. The uneven, nonsensical reimbursement system. The cost of running a business (most surgeons are in private practice and, therefore, running a business). Practicing surgery today is much more than being a surgical professional—and a lot of it is stuff we never bargained for in medical school.

This book is my story, and my examination of a unique occupation—truly a "calling" in many respects—that requires years of arduous training, followed by years of arduous work, where fatigue and malpractice lawyers take turns attempting to distract us from the job at hand: a person's life.

What in the world possessed me to write this book? This question has floated through my mind ever since the idea was conceived. Even now, I ask myself. I ask, yet I continue to write. I write because I seek the truth about myself and about those I have affected, for better or worse. I believe the truth will set you free. It has for me.

Paul A. Ruggieri, M.D., F.A.C.S.
March 2011

Chapter 1

///

The Making of a Surgeon

The first two fingers of my right hand were rigid with fear, frozen in position. My crisp white doctor's coat was beginning to wilt from the sweat racing down my back. The tension in the room was rising. I simply had no idea what my next move should be. *Stay calm, keep it together, and listen,* I told myself. *Just focus on the task in front of you.*

I was a newly minted third-year medical student, officially "licensed" to lay my hands on patients. It was about time. We were all champing at the bit. With just two years of medical classes behind me, I was ready to be a doctor and, ultimately (I hoped), a surgeon. I was looking forward to touching a live human being. The surgeon in me was looking forward to making that first scalpel cut. Today was a day for touching; cutting would have to wait.

1

All of us had been prepped, briefly, by our professors for this "special" day, but nothing too specific had been shared. The vagueness seemed a little odd, but we were there to learn, not question. In retrospect, seeing how a person handles the unknown was (and still is) part of the making of a surgeon. Thinking quickly and making judgments under stress—with very little time to evaluate—are the hallmarks of a surgeon's daily life.

Most of my classmates were lined up with me. We stood outside two doorways, like city workers waiting to get into a deli at lunchtime. There were no pastrami sandwiches, however, on the other side of those doors. The rooms ahead of us were filled with operating room tables and live patients. As I stepped into the first room, lunch was the furthest thing from my mind.

The "task" in front of me, on which I was trying to focus, was a female "model" hired by the medical school. I could feel the tension in my fingers migrating into my arm, neck, back, and legs. *How in the world is this going to make me into a surgeon?* I thought, trying to justify my insecurity. *I don't need this.* I struggled to avoid eye contact with her.

"Hello, Dr. Ruggieri." I could smell the whiff of sarcasm in her voice. I always hated being called this, knowing that in reality I was one step ahead of a glorified graduate student. The calmness of the female voice directly in front of me jerked my ego back into place. "My name is Roxanne. Please move your fingers in deeper and gently place your left hand here." She grabbed my stiff left hand and placed it just above her pubic bone. I was unable to utter a word. "Now, sweep your right two fingers to the left and simultaneously put pressure down with your left hand. Can you feel my right ovary as it moves across your fingers?" I nodded sheepishly, stuttering something resembling a yes. Hell, in this situation, I wasn't going to feel an ovary if it hit me between the eyes. I tried to focus, tried to fight off the mental and physical distractions. The whole thing felt like a bowl of warm jelly.

This was my first clinical pelvic exam and, in my mind, I was failing miserably. The situation was out of my control. My fingers, arm, and neck were so tensed up I would have admitted to anything to get the "exercise" over with. We were eyeball to eyeball, my right hand deep in dark territory. Her legs were in stirrups, while mine were about to buckle. Her confident voice was trying to educate me while I was privately praying for a power failure. I was experiencing very mixed emotions. Just three years earlier I had been working as an ironworker, saving money to attend medical school. My hands were constantly being traumatized by wire and metal rods. Interestingly enough, the guys I worked with then regularly discussed their "examination" of various parts of the female anatomy. Although, their "exams" were in a somewhat different setting from the one I now found myself in. Now, my gloved hands probed into a living stranger's body while a voice directed their every move. It was all very surreal. I felt uncomfortable on several levels. For one thing, my fingers were stuck in someone's vagina and I didn't know what the hell I was feeling. For another, I was shy about where I was, because my overall experience with women was not as robust as that of some of my colleagues.

When Roxanne was through with me, I was allowed to move

on to the next clinical lesson: a male model, in an adjacent room, ready to educate me in the art of . . . well, you get the picture. Needless to say, I was traumatized by the entire experience and continue to have occasional flashbacks when I see a stirrup in the operating room.

When it was over, I had learned two valuable lessons. The first: I was not going to be a gynecologist. This was one part of a person's anatomy I did not want to make a career out of. The second, and more important, was being introduced to the milieu of a surgeon's daily life: dealing quickly with the unknown, facing one's insecurities and even, sometimes, one's humility. Looking back, I believe the entire experience was orchestrated not to fine-tune our clinical ability to perform an adequate pelvic examination—it was, rather, the first of many lessons that would introduce us to the world of clinical stress, assessing the unknown and reacting to the best of our abilities. The making of a surgeon had begun.

///

We had named her Tilly. She reminded one of the members in our group of his Aunt Tilly, so the name stuck. Welcome to the family.

Tilly was our dissecting cadaver, introduced to us during the first week of anatomy class, a woman whom we would get to know intimately over the next five months. A woman who, even in death, would contribute to the making of several surgeons throughout the weeks ahead.

She was probably in her early seventies when she died,

willingly donating her body to the future doctors of the world. We knew nothing else about her. We did not know how she died, where she came from, or who her family was. Her face and body appeared well-preserved, gold fillings and purple nail polish neatly intact (the nail polish was a little freaky). If it weren't for the lingering odor of formaldehyde, we would not have been surprised if she sat up suddenly and offered us some fresh baked cookies.

Yet despite these aspects of parts of her physical appearance, she did not *look* human. She was not real. How could she be? Her face was constantly covered, while the rest of her body was completely exposed. Our work began on her torso, moved to her extremities, and reserved her face for last. We had no human connection to her, nothing to prevent us from calmly carving her up like a turkey, body part by body part, over the next five months. It was all in the name of learning, of course. The six of us were on a mission to learn human anatomy at any cost.

In addition to mastering the rigors of the class work, first-year human anatomy forced many in my group to face previously foreign thoughts and emotions. Before meeting Tilly, I had never been personally introduced to death. Up to that point, death had not touched my life. Now, as soon as the sheets were removed, I was face-to-face with death and did not have the experience or desire to process its meaning. Who does? None of us welcomes death or is eager to face it, no matter how it presents itself.

To me, Tilly was not dead. She was very much alive and helping me become a surgeon every day during anatomy class. Some of us talked to Tilly during our dissections. In essence, she truly was a member of our family: six medical students trying to survive anatomy class. We spent so much time with her that she was even introduced to our extended family. One of my best friends today was a classmate I met during the first days of medical school. We were both assigned to Tilly, brought together by the first initial of our last names. Steven Rockoff (now a practicing urologist—with that name, what else could he be?) was one of my dissecting partners, one of the group of six. He became so enamored with Tilly that one evening he brought the woman he hoped to make his wife to meet her.

They made plans to meet in the cadaver lab late one Friday night, where Rock planned to impress her with his lab coat and knowledge of human anatomy. It was one of their first dates. Elaine was a nursing student at Georgetown University, and "Rock" was very interested in expanding their relationship. I'm not sure Elaine was as eager. As medical students, we were at the bottom of the dating food chain. Working nurses would not give us the time of day while we were in the hospital. Our earning potential was just a faint silhouette on the career horizon. Plus, they were smarter than we were. Surgical residents, on the other hand, were the hunted ones. They were closer to realizing their earning potential, closer to the real world. So with this reality, we focused on impressing nursing students. Rock's cadaver date was a success (in thanks, partly, to Tilly), and Rock and Elaine married several years later. They have now been together for the better part of twenty years and have four beautiful children. Even in death, Tilly was alive, bringing people together.

What does medical school have to do with the making of a

surgeon? Not a whole lot. Yes, it is a place to start, a place that inspires you to study hard. Yet in many ways you are coddled, protected from any real responsibility. It is truly just the *beginning* of a unique journey that takes a lifetime to complete. I was very happy to be there, because I failed to get into medical school the first time around. That wasn't the first time I had experienced failure, and it was not going to be the last. Experiencing failure along with success helps a developing surgeon stay grounded and humble—especially important in light of the pedestal on which society soon places you.

Medical school provided me with the basics of human anatomy, physiology, and clinical diagnosis. I was ready to move on to the next level of training and responsibility for patients. It also provided me with a lot of financial debt. (Years later, I would find out how real both the debt and the responsibility were.) Similar to surgical residency, medical school was actually a test of students' mental ability to adjust to the mass of information thrown at them. The medical school gods wanted to see who would thrive in this environment of information overload. Although there was much more at stake during surgical training—such as people's lives—medical school was a contest of survival of the fittest. Not everyone made it; there were those who survived and those who were left behind.

Even in the clinical years—learning how to interview patients, diagnose disease, and care for patients—the curriculum was, indirectly, herding us into the specialties we would eventually choose. I wanted to be a surgeon. This fact was clear to me on the first day of medical school. I wanted to use my hands to cut out disease. I wanted to use my mental and physical skills to get instant results with patients. I could see that surgeons were independent thinkers, relying only on themselves for success. Surgeons were gods. They also appeared to make a lot of money. I wanted to be a surgeon. It was during this year that we were exposed to every specialty in clinical medicine, as varied as ob/gyn (which I immediately eliminated after the "teaching" pelvic exam) and psychiatry. During each specialty rotation, we clung to the coattails of residents in training, gaining experience in a different section of clinical medicine each time. The hope was that these experiences would trigger a career choice. I still recall one clinical rotation that triggered some serious exercise.

I was rotating through psychiatry with my good friend Rock when one of our patients escaped the ward. Rock had just finished interviewing the patient. I am not sure what Rock had said but the patient took off, running into the parking lot, screaming to the high heavens. Like the would-be surgeons we aspired to be, we had to act—and quickly. We took to the chase. Rock made the initial tackle and I subsequently piled on. It was a beautiful thing, white coats, dirt, and a psych patient all in a scrum. We returned the patient to the ward, hailed by the nurses as the conquering heroes. Our physician psychiatry mentor, however, was not pleased. "What the hell were you guys thinking? You're medical students, for God's sake." She never liked us, from the beginning.

"Well, Dr. Bernards," I paused, "we want to be surgeons, so we reacted like surgeons." That was the wrong thing to say. Our short career as budding psychiatrists ended on the pavement in the parking lot.

The making of a surgeon *really* began during my surgical rotation as a third-year medical student. It was during these six weeks of information overload, long hours in the operating room, and time "on call" (caring for patients while the rest of the world slept) that a career started to take shape. It was during this rotation that I got an addictive sweet taste of being a surgeon. As on the other rotations, I gained my experience by following the surgical residents around, begging for responsibility, which was given in very small increments and at their discretion. By the end of my surgical experience during medical school, I could barely tie a knot and would have been hard-pressed to dissect my way out of a paper bag. There simply was not enough practice to acquire those skills. But the truth was I didn't need them yet. Those lessons were ahead of me.

Surgeons are independent doers, ready to act. They prefer not to ask for help, thank you, or to place trust in much outside their own abilities. They work hard, expect perfection, and do not accept excuses. To the residents, some surgeon mentors were decent human beings; others were tyrants. Personalities aside, the central fact was this: Surgeons use their hard-earned physical skills to get results in the operating room (or create their own problems). They rely on themselves for success or failure. They are the captains of their ships. They do not need or want to rely on medication or another person to improve the quality of a patient's life. Surgery is a specialty of instant gratification, for patient and surgeon alike.

As a third-year medical student, I was in awe of the surgical residents' stamina and ability to function on very little sleep.

This was what I wanted to be. I wasn't interested in caring for the "whole" person. I did not have the personality—or the brains, for that matter. I greatly admire my internal medicine colleagues for their thinking abilities in the face of so much information to process. I wanted to be the type of doctor who came in immediately and, despite adversity, made a perfect mark, soon after which I'd leave and forever be remembered as the conquering hero. It would be a straightforward and satisfying career. Little did I know what lay beyond the protective walls of medical school.

I was a first-year surgical intern at a major teaching surgical program in the Midwest, fueled by coffee and motivated by the desire to be the best. It was twenty-four hours on and twenty-four hours off in the emergency room for six weeks. I mostly slept during the twenty-four hours off, getting up long enough to shower, shave, get some exercise, and eat. Meaningful relationships? Forget about it. Sex was a distraction and out of the question.

As a surgical intern in the emergency room, I was the first line of surgical defense. The first to lay hands on any surgical patient that entered. There was no one with me, no one to offer support. I was it. On one of my first days, I noticed the multitude of *medical* interns scurrying about, all helping one another in caring for the "medical" patients that came in. There was plenty of support on the medical side, but I, the surgical intern, was an island unto myself.

If someone came through the emergency room with a surgical problem, I was the one to make the diagnosis. I was the one to call the surgical team if an operation was needed. I dared not ask for help during the process of evaluating someone; it would have been considered a sign of weakness. It was never a spoken rule, but showing weakness of any kind was out of the question. It wasn't an option. Everyone who wanted to advance understood it.

Mr. Williams was one of the first patients to test my young clinical skills in surgical diagnosis when he checked in with the complaint of abdominal pain.

"Doc, I have this pain down here in my pelvis and it's getting worse."

I quickly looked him over, examined his abdomen, and silently reviewed what the leading diagnoses could be. *Appendicitis? Maybe. Diverticulitis? Possibly. Could be a hernia.* I kept whispering to myself, going over the differential diagnosis of abdominal pain I had learned as a medical student. "I think we need to get an x-ray of your abdomen and take it from there," I told him. I was eager to make the correct diagnosis and serve the guy up to my chief resident for an operation.

The man silently agreed. I sensed there was more to his story but just didn't have time to pursue it—another patient had just checked in with a laceration to his forehead. He was bleeding all over the floor and needed quick attention. I quickly stemmed the bleeding with some pressure and, with the help of a nurse, sutured the man up and sent him packing. I then made my way over to the x-ray department to look at Mr. Williams's abdominal films.

"Mr. Williams," I said as I slapped his x-rays up onto the lighted board in the room. He was pacing. "Can you tell me what this thing is and how in the world it got there?" I pointed to a buoy-shaped bottle deep in his pelvis.

"Listen, Doc, it was an accident." He was looking at the floor, shuffling. "I was taking a shower. Next thing I know, I slipped on a bar of soap and landed right on this bottle of cologne, you know, Old Spice cologne. The thing went right up my butt." He was unable to look up.

I was speechless and not interested in finding out more. I did not want to know. In many cases, I don't want to know the specifics. Just show me where the problem is so I can fix it, remove it, rearrange it, drain it, or pass you on to someone else. All those fancy surgical diagnoses swimming around in my head were blown out of the water. Forget about impressing my chief resident with a methodical approach to a working diagnosis of acute appendicitis. All I'd had to do was examine the man's rectum and my *fingers* would have made the diagnosis. The man had a bottle of Old Spice cologne stuck up his rectum. This was his diagnosis— not standard reading in any surgical text I had come across.

Out of embarrassment, and disgust at myself, I just motioned for him to turn around and drop his pants. My gloved, lubricated finger was not going anywhere. Clink. "Yes, sir. You definitely have a bottle wedged up there. And it's not coming out. We will have to put you to sleep in the operating room to get this thing out." He didn't care and I was through caring. Problem identified and soon to be solved. He just wanted it out and I needed to attend to the next patient, and the next patient, and the next.

During the next six weeks of this surgical rite of passage, I inadvertently stuck myself twice with contaminated needles, briefly nodded off in the middle of suturing a leg laceration, accidentally punctured a guy's femoral artery while trying to draw some blood, and broke up a fight between the family members of a guy who came in with a stab wound to the abdomen. I was slugged in the head by a delirious patient in an alcoholic rage, spat upon, coughed on, vomited on, farted on, bled on, and mistaken for an orderly. My patients were kind enough to introduce me to maggots, leeches, roaches, ants, and an array of kitchen utensils lodged in the most unsuspecting places on their body. All I wanted to do was survive.

How does the training system in this country turn a raw medical school graduate, with few or no surgical abilities, into the masked surgeon you see in the operating room before you are put to sleep? The making of a surgeon during surgical training is a high-stakes survival test, not necessarily mastered by the brightest but rather by those who are driven, who find a way to get things done in the face of emotional and physical adversity. It is an experience that brings out the best (and the worst) in everyone involved. You are cast into a chaotic environment that initially breaks you down to a hollow, humble shell. Then, if you progress, the shell is gradually filled in with morsels of self-confidence, patient-care knowledge, and hands-on surgical experience. If you qualify, the system embraces you with open arms, encouraging you on with glimpses of the dazzling trappings of success that await. Once you are part of this exclusive club, the rules, indoctrinations, and peer pressure shape your thinking, hold you hostage, and, finally, steady your hand with each stroke of the scalpel.

Surgical training is called "training" for a reason. You are there to learn how to operate competently and care for the surgical patient. Like most training programs then and now, the premise is to expose you to more responsibility each year while you work, supervised by those above you. With each passing year, I was given more responsibility to operate independently but always under the watchful eyes of my peers. Because we were learning "on the job," mistakes did occur. Any surgeon can regale you with accounts of surgical mishaps during training days: operating on the wrong body part, inadvertently cutting into the wrong organs. To this day, I can still see the faces of the patients who died while under my care, patients I failed. Finally, after five years of intense training, I had amassed the skills to operate and care for patients independently.

I can describe, with one word, the driving force behind my five years of surgical training: *fear.* My training program was ruled by a chairman who had roots in the dark ages of the old surgical guard. Up until the late 1990s, many of the top general surgical training programs still resembled those from the old school of thinking in their structure, competitiveness, and abusiveness. These programs were brutal in their workload, often bringing you to the brink of mental and physical exhaustion. One of the brightest and strongest in my class was brought to his knees by the pressure while on call in the cardiac surgery service. This resident seemed indestructible, or so we all thought. One night, one of the nurses paged him. No answer. He was eventually found in a fetal position in the call room, useless to anyone. He ended up becoming an anesthesiologist and lived happily ever after. If it didn't kill you, surgical training made you stronger.

Times have changed for residents. It all changed because of the unexpected death of a patient in a New York city hospital in 1984. Libby Zion walked into an emergency room, ill and looking for care. She left in a body bag. Her father was a high-profile citizen of the city and would not accept the initial explanations of her death as fact. At his legal and political urging, state authorities investigated the details of Libby's care (helped along by his vigorous lawsuit). In the end, the legal case and investigation uncovered what most residents already knew and lived.

Libby Zion's death exposed the exhaustive pressures and lack of supervision that were the norm in many training programs, both of which increased the potential for serious mistakes, and led to reforms including the number of hours residents could work continuously without sleep. Libby's death ultimately closed the door on residencies rooted in the old way of thinking: "Survive no matter what the circumstances." Initially, in the late 1980s, the reforms instituted in New York first trickled into the *medical* residencies only. It wasn't until the publication of the landmark paper *To Err Is Human*—which concluded that 44,000 to 98,000 people died in hospitals each year from medical errors—that these reforms found their way to the *surgical* teaching programs in this country as well.

In July 2003, all surgical residencies in this country changed, for better or worse, depending on whom you talk to. I was a product of the old school of training, taking whatever fatigue, abuse, and work came my way. I learned how to keep moving forward despite the unrealistic workload and constant sleep deprivation. I learned to operate mainly from the residents above me, not directly from mentors. Yes, mistakes were made because of fatigue and inexperience. Yet the system worked for me and many of my colleagues. It forced me to dig deep and find out what I was made of, especially when blood was squirting off the table. Those experiences made me the surgeon I am today. I would not have wanted it any other way. I salivated when a trauma patient arrived in the middle of the night, knowing I would get the chance to operate despite the exhaustion and early-morning hour. This would be *my* case. These patients would be *my* responsibility. While the rest of the world slept, I was gaining invaluable experience.

I do have some misgivings about the surgeons coming out of training today. I have concerns regarding their overall operative experience, given today's strict enforcement of the eighty-hours-a-week work rule. Most of my best (and worst) work was done in the 100th or 120th hour of the workweek. The best work was gratifying; the worst work was at least character-building. The jury is still out regarding the experience of surgeons coming out of training today; as a result of the reforms, are they less experienced than the generation before? Surgical residents have a better quality of life today. No doubt. But the real question is: *Are they as competent to operate as the mentors who trained them?*

I ask this with the benefit of having spent three years on active duty as a general surgeon in the U.S. Army. Those three years presented me with the opportunity to perfect my diagnostic and surgical skills. They also allowed me to decompress and rid myself of all the mental baggage carried from residency. As a surgeon in the military, stationed on a base in the middle of

Cajun swamp country, I quickly learned to operate efficiently by myself. I also had to learn how to stay out of trouble in the operating room and deal with any mistakes I created. As a surgeon in the military, I had no one around to bail me out.

During my training experience, the men who ruled surgical residency programs were giants in the surgical lore, and most ruled with a strong fist. That was how *they* had been taught. Their past torments were, in turn, passed down to us. They were gods in their kingdom and were not eager to give up their surgical secrets without a mental and physical price. They had the power to do whatever they wanted with you. To them, you were privileged to be abused in their programs. These were not humane, friendly programs but brutal tests of stamina and determination. In addition to the inhumane workload and hours, often you had to put up with intense verbal abuse from those trying to shape you. Everything was your fault, regardless of the circumstances. If your mentor surgeon was operating and cut into the wrong artery, it was your fault for not giving him or her a warning. If a patient under your care had a setback on the floor, guess whose fault it was. You just had to let the shit bounce off and adapt to every situation. The fear vultures were always hovering.

///

"Hey, Dr. Ruggieri. Welcome back. We missed you. Did you miss us?" Cathie was the first to greet me as I returned to the S.I.C.U. (surgical intensive care unit) during the second year of my residency.

"Oh yes, just like I miss a thrombosed hemorrhoid." I was kidding, but deep down I knew what the next six weeks would bring. "You and I are going to get to know each other very well this time." Surgical intensive care patients require vigilant, around-the-clock care. I shook my finger. "No sex, sleep, or exercise for me the next six weeks."

"Doctor, I am looking forward to our time together." She was flirting. She knew she owned me for six weeks. During my time as a surgical resident, my entire social, personal, political, financial, and religious life unfolded in the hospital. The women I met and slept with were all people working in the hospital. Cathie was a smart, dedicated, and attractive nurse who was a veteran of the S.I.C.U. She knew a hell of a lot more than we lowly residents when it came to taking care of critically ill patients. I knew it. I respected her ability to recognize problems and "act first, ask permission later." As a resident, I dared not insult Cathie with my "I'm the doctor and you're the nurse" routine because she was the actual doctor and I felt like the nurse. She could make my life tolerable or miserable. As luck would have it, Cathie saved my ass many times during my stay in the S.I.C.U. by alerting me to problems in patients before they got out of hand. During one of my first nights on call, Cathie sensed that her patient, a fresh postoperative colon resection, was bleeding internally. His vital signs were going the wrong way. Something was not right. It was three in the morning and I was dead to the world, asleep in the call room. She quickly informed me that the patient was bleeding. Several blood tests later, her patient was whisked back to the operating room to stop intra-abdominal bleeding.

Some weeks later, I was introduced to Jane late one night during my S.I.C.U. rotation. Jane was a young, healthy woman about to give birth to her first child. She and her husband were living the American dream. I, too, was living the American dream. I was a tired, out-of-shape resident who had just finished a Twinkie (my go-to late-night snack in those days) and was trying to catch ten minutes of sleep in a chair in a dark corner. Toward the end of her pregnancy, Jane's liver started to fail acutely. She was lucky enough to deliver her baby before it completely shut down, threatening her life. This was a rare and serious medical phenomenon; most patients die without ever seeing the newborn. She was critically ill and on life support when I met her in the intensive care unit. Jane hadn't seen her baby, lapsing into a coma immediately after giving birth. Her only hope was a liver transplant to reverse the downward spiral of her diseased physiology. Someone, somewhere, had to die soon so Jane could live to be a mother. Time was of the essence.

"Shit, this is going to be a long night." I could barely lift my eyelids. There was half a Twinkie wedged in my pants. I quickly got up and moved toward the room, watching the nurses plug tubes, wires, and catheters into their homes. Her entire body was full of fluid, her face yellow as a squash. For a second, I let my emotional guard down, wondering how the forces of the universe could turn such an amazing event, the birth of child, into the brink of death for the woman who bore it.

"Ruggieri, Dr. Harrison on the phone." Two seconds had passed. Here we go. Dr. Harrison was a new liver transplant surgeon whose reputation evoked fear in every resident who worked under him, including me. He was a little guy with big eyes and a frightening bark. He was known to work harder than any resident. He was also a genius, but his temper eruptions were beginning to gain a reputation throughout the hospital.

"Paul," he said, his voice psychotically calm, "we have a liver for Jane. I will be in touch after the transplant."

"Yes, sir." That was all I could muster. Click. I went back to look at Jane. I could not recognize a mother in her bed.

Once the transplant surgery was over, all I could envision was the next ten hours of no rest while trying to keep Jane alive. I was dreading Dr. Harrison breathing down my neck, calling every hour for an update. There was much at stake here, for Dr. Harrison, for me, and most of all for Jane. This was his first liver transplant operation at the university, so I knew he would be all over it, and me. If this woman's new liver failed because of something I did not recognize while caring for her in the intensive care unit, I would need intensive care. Dr. Harrison's professional reputation was at stake along with my job. Everyone was watching this one.

Jane's surgery went well, and she returned to the S.I.C.U. The next twelve hours were critical in detecting problems with her new liver, problems that would be correctable *if* recognized in time. Every hour, on the hour, Dr. Harrison would call for an update on how well her liver was functioning. It was three A.M. At this point, Jane was not a human being to me, lying there with tubes exiting every orifice. She was a newly transplanted liver, an organ I had to keep functioning so it could eventually restore her motherhood. I had a job to do. I had to shut the window on any emotional interference. I could not let Dr. Harrison down. I could not let the surgical ghosts of my past down.

That night turned into several weeks in the surgical intensive care unit, and Jane's newly transplanted liver responded beautifully. She eventually left the hospital with her newborn and continued living the American dream. I survived my S.I.C.U. rotation and moved on to the next year of residency. Several years ago I came across an alumni article with a picture of Jane and her family, heralding a milestone anniversary of her liver transplant success. She was the most beautiful liver I had ever seen.

/ / /

As the rest of my surgical training unfolded, I continued to gain more operating experience and began to feel, finally, like a real surgeon. Each year of training continued to bring new operative successes and failures. One of the early operations I was privileged to perform was a leg amputation. The operation itself is relatively primitive, not far removed from the days of the "butcher surgeons." Primitive, yes, but it was a chance for me to cut. The freaky aspect of this operation came when it was time to hand off the amputated leg to the nurse. For a second, you realize you have just cut off someone's leg, a leg that has walked places and worn shoes. On my first leg amputation, the handoff did not go well.

"Nurse, bag please." I tried to sound like a real surgeon despite this being one of my first solo operations. As I lifted the newly severed leg off the table, the reality of the moment hit me. I had willingly cut a man's leg off. My hands were shaking and

I suddenly lost my balance. *Son of a bitch.* The leg missed the open bag and landed on the floor with a thud, a squirt of blood spitting out from the cut femoral artery. The operating room went silent.

"Sorry about that." It was all I could muster.

"Well, aren't you going to pick it up?" The operating room nurse's eyes glared at me. "Do you think it is going to jump in there by itself? Please. Pick up your mess."

I sheepishly bent down, picked up the leg, and deposited it into the bag.

///

In my final year as a chief resident, I was operating independently under the "supervision" of my mentors, gearing up for the outside world. During the day, supervisors were all around us. In the middle of the night, good luck trying to get one of them to come in. It often took an act of God to make this happen. Again, time and energy were scarce commodities, and emotions had to be buried. There was never any time or energy to dwell on anything but the tasks directly in front of you. Displaying emotions was a sign of weakness. I often prayed to get through the program without directly contributing to the death of a patient, especially as a chief resident. If a patient died on your service as a chief resident, for whatever reason, it was your fault. You were accountable for it and had to explain yourself to the chairman. It was never a pleasant experience to get called to the chairman's office. He didn't say much. He didn't have to. The stare was enough to wreak havoc on your intestinal tract.

The man was intense. In my position as chief resident, one of my main goals was to keep the sick patients I had inherited from the previous chief alive long enough to pass them on to the next chief. Dying was not an option.

Complications after surgery, or a death, were deemed personal failures and had to be explained, often in an arena of your peers. Throughout the rest of my training, I continued to meet interesting mentors who guided my surgical hand. These "teachers" came in all shapes, sizes, egos, and skills. There was the thoracic surgeon who, after removing a cancerous lung (caused by smoking) from a patient, would go into the back room and calmly light up a Marlboro. That was inspiring. I have always wondered what he died of. There was the surgeon who was board certified in four subspecialties. The man was brilliant, a true jack-of-all-surgical-trades. He also ran a research lab. He made it all look so easy. I hated guys who made it look easy.

There was the "Puerto Rican hurricane," a vascular surgeon who would have several operating rooms going at the same time. He was built like a hurricane: broad shoulders, strong hands, and always in the eye of the operating room storm. He would sweep in, guide the chief resident through the critical part of the operation, then move on to the next room. The man could operate incredibly well under pressure. We all shook our heads in amazement. Several other mentors, to this day, resurface in my mind from time to time. On the nightmare side, there was Dr. Miles Wilson, the Dr. Jekyll and Mr. Hyde of transplant surgery. Outside the operating room, Dr. Wilson morphed into a likable, "I want to be your friend!" teacher who was very concerned about your surgical experience.

Inside the operating room, his constant barrage of insults, F-bombs, and belittling tirades was relentless. To me, the man was a coward, taking out his personal insecurities on the sheep around him while using the secrecy of the operating room as cover. The surprise was that he had superb operating skills. To this day, I am not sure what could have caused such a hideous transformation once he stepped inside the operating room. My guess is he trained under one of the biggest (and smartest) dogs in transplant surgery, who probably barked, spat, drooled, and farted all over him in the operating room. He was now in a position to do the same.

Dr. Clifford Peters, a cardiac surgery fellow, was, to all of us, one of Mt. Olympus's surgical gods. He was completing an additional training in heart surgery when I arrived on his service as a lowly resident. Cliff was a brilliant, handsome, chiseled, soon-to-be heart surgeon who had the bravado, the ego, and the skills to master any situation in life. Often he taught those who were supposedly teaching him how to get out of trouble in the operating room. He knew he was better than several of his mentors and was not afraid to show it if a patient's life hung in the balance. Cliff was born to be a heart surgeon. God had placed him on this earth to fix or replace broken hearts. He was untouchable and everyone knew it. In our eyes, he was the John Wayne of heart surgery. Cliff could have been a movie star, a C.E.O., a professional athlete, or a general in the military. The man was a leader, a teacher, an author, and an inspiration. A tribute to his greatness was his ability to teach, often getting the best out of us without having to beat us like dogs. We all aspired to be Dr. Clifford Peters. None of us would ever come close.

After he completed his training to start a cardiac transplant program in New Orleans, I lost track of his career for many years. It was not until a short time ago that I was updated on Cliff's extraordinary life and unexpected death. While reminiscing with friends over dinner on a trip to New Orleans, I learned that Cliff had succumbed to a rare form of leukemia. I was shaken to the core by the news. Cliff was invincible, or so we thought. In our jobs, death is around all of us every day, but as surgeons we think we are immune to it. Perhaps the greatest irony of Cliff's illness was that it presented as a heart-related problem, the very organ he had mastered. It was only later that testing revealed a very aggressive form of leukemia as the underlying cause of his initial heart ailment. With his talents as a cardiac transplant surgeon, Cliff had reveled in keeping death's shadow from darkening so many lives. But when the gods called, he could not save his own. He was only a few years older than I when he passed, leaving behind a wife, children, and many grateful patients. Surgical gods are never supposed to die.

///

"I would qualify him as a safe surgeon." Those are the words I remember most from my final evaluation as chief surgical resident. As lackluster as this commentary seemed to me at the time, I was not going to let it sour the last moments of an extraordinary experience—my surgical training.

No, I was not a rising star, someone who had been born with exceptionally gifted hands. I hadn't graduated at the top of my medical school class. (I was somewhere in the middle.) I wasn't a stellar resident who could quote journal articles while operating deep inside someone's abdomen. Yes, I had been able to make the transformation from a raw surgical intern (unable to tie a knot efficiently) to an independently operating surgeon. When had this transformation occurred? It is difficult to pinpoint. At some moment during my last year, I had an epiphany. It was at that moment I realized, *I can do this.*

"Safe surgeon." My surgical training was over. Behind me, five years of sweat, blood, fatigue, successes, failures, surgical misadventures, and death. Ahead of me, I could expect more of the same. The difference: responsibility. I alone would now be accountable for my successes, complications, and failures—no one else. I was still a work in progress, still in need of grooming by the real world of surgical practice. For now, though, I had been judged to be a "safe" surgeon, safe enough to perform surgery without the supervision of a mentor. But was I? Yes, I had the knowledge to diagnose many surgical diseases and prepare patients for surgery. Yes, I was technically capable of removing a section of cancerous colon, suturing up holes in a shot-up intestine at three in the morning, or repairing complex abdominal wall hernias. Yes, I could confidently guide a patient through postoperative recovery. Yes, I could stay up for several days without sleep and still function or stand in the same spot for hours, operating and holding off a full bladder.

Over the last five years, I had labored to learn the skills of surgery and earned the right to move on. But what had I truly learned about myself? Would I continue to view my patients as just a gallbladder, a colon, a thyroid, or a hernia, or would I view each one now as a whole person with a surgical problem? Would I be able to exhibit compassion on a daily basis? Had I really learned how to operate without the safety net of a mentor? Would I have the mental calmness to get myself out of trouble, trouble I created, in the operating room? How would I feel about my first serious complication, or the first death of a patient caused by a misjudgment? Would I be able to take full responsibility and be truthful about the circumstances? Would I be able to know my own limitations and not let pride or money control the scalpel in my hand? Would I be open to constructive criticism, accept blame, and not let my ego's protective shield cover me. How would I react the first time I got sued?

The making of a surgeon had begun.

Chapter 2

///

Are Surgeons Human?

I wanted him to die. I really did. I was hoping his heart's pumping action would just stop. I was hoping he would never make it to the operating room.

The man had just gone on a shooting rampage in the local courtroom, distraught over an ugly ongoing divorce. He had expressed his festering anger by emptying several rounds from a .38-caliber handgun into his wife, his wife's divorce lawyer, and other colleagues during legal proceedings in the courtroom. He had only wounded his wife with the first shot to her neck. She was still breathing, gasping for life, when he calmly walked around the table. He slowly squatted next to her and placed the gun to her head. The second shot killed her instantly.

I was the chief resident on the trauma service on duty in the hospital when the shooter arrived with nine bullet wounds, care of the local police. If the man needed to go to surgery, I was the one to take him. Minutes before his arrival, my team and I were alerted to the incoming carnage. I was pacing back and forth. The shooter arrived in the main trauma room. "Shot nine times, twice in the head, and you are still breathing," I whispered under my breath as I approached him. His victims arrived several minutes later. The shooter was the most critically ill of those who were brought to the emergency room that night. The irony: *He* had to go to the operating room first. He had to be saved first. Blood from his head wounds was beginning to accumulate on the floor. It was a steady drip, drip, drip.

"You son of a bitch . . ." I mumbled. He would not meet my gaze. *Why don't you save the families of the victims a lot of grief, save the taxpayers a lot of money, and allow me to sleep tonight by just checking out?* For a moment, I let my emotions get the best of me. For a moment, I was filled with rage. For a moment, I wanted the shooter to die. He did not deserve the extraordinary efforts the surgical team would soon deploy to keep him alive that night. He did not deserve a trial, given the obvious weight of his guilt. It was all black-and-white to me.

"Dr. Ruggieri." The trauma nurse's voice jolted me back to my reality, the reality of what I was trained to do. "The operating room is ready. Any other orders before we get this guy up there?" Fortunately for him, my profession does not discriminate at death's door. To me, the operating room is considered the great equalizer. All who pass through those doors are one and the same. In the end, there was no moral dilemma; he was gravely injured and I could help him.

"No, Nurse. Just get him upstairs quickly." It was time to save a life.

Once I had his abdomen open in the operating room, nothing beyond repairing the holes in his intestine and repairing damaged blood vessels mattered. "Nurse, clamp now!" A jet of blood rose up and was heading for my right eye. It always does. I turned my head just in time. "Get this guy off me." I needed a wipe.

With each saving stitch, I wasn't saving the life of a murderer. I was doing what I was trained to do. I did not give a shit about his life before he entered my operating room. He was just a trauma case to me, nothing more. The circumstances surrounding his entrance to my "office" did not matter now. It did not matter how many people he might have killed. I needed to use the powers bestowed by my surgical mentors to get him off the table alive. I did not want him dying on the table, because it would lead to a messy situation. There would be too many questions to answer and too much paperwork to fill out. Once under anesthesia, with the body part I needed to cut into draped off, he was just like all the others who came before him, despite his heinous crime. At that moment, to me he was several feet of shot-up intestine, damaged blood vessels, a shot-up liver, and a half-dollar-sized opening in his stomach. He was no different than the gallbladder I removed on Mr. Barber yesterday or the colon cancer I resected on Mrs. Johnson last week.

Once a patient is on the operating room table asleep, draped off, and ready to be cut open, I do not consider him or her human. All I see is a diseased appendix, a cancerous thyroid mass, a hernia, or an inflamed gallbladder. Yes, I realize there is a life, a soul, attached to these organs. In order to do my job effectively, however, I cannot allow it to be a distraction. There are no "feelings" inside the operating room, no time for reflection. Here, I do not consider myself human. At that moment, I am devoid of any feelings for the patient. I am a robot, blocking out any outside interferences. I have to be methodical, carrying out precise surgical maneuvers, removing, rearranging, or patching up whatever brought me there. In my work as a general surgeon, this is what I am and what I see. Orthopedic surgeons may see a diseased hip that needs to be replaced. Cardiac surgeons may see a diseased coronary vessel in need of bypassing. Gynecologists may see a diseased uterus that needs to go.

It is only after the shooter is made whole again that the despicable human being who took away a life surfaces. Just as it is only after Mr. Barber's gallbladder has been removed that he is again the local banker whose son is the star quarterback for the football team. After it was all over, the shooter survived his wounds, was tried and convicted in a court of law, and, ultimately, was sentenced to death.

This violent episode was the first time I had to struggle with conflicting emotions between what my heart desired and what my training directed my hand to do. It would not be the last. There would be more critically ill patients after the shooter who would force me to revisit the conflict between the emotions in my heart and the scalpel in my hand.

The rigors of surgical training are not conducive to the exploring of human emotions. There was no energy left, no emotional reservoir to begin to dwell on the unique emotions attached to the life-and-death situations in training. I do vividly remember the first patient who died on the operating room table in a case in which I was the chief surgeon. It was during my last year of training. I remember, not because of the emotional impact it made but because of how quickly death arrived. The patient had arrived in the middle of the night. (They all do.) He was another gunshot victim of an ongoing drug war. Upon seeing him in the emergency room, the junior resident and I knew he was doomed. He was the victim of multiple gunshot wounds to the abdomen, a casualty of his profession. His blood pressure was dropping like a stone because of internal hemorrhaging. He needed to get to the operating room quickly or he soon would be another anonymous statistic. Despite our efforts, the operation was an exercise in futility. As soon as we opened his abdomen, blood mixed with stool gushed forth from his injuries and spilled off the operating room table.

"Shit, I knew I should have double booted. I just bought these shoes and now look at them." There is a funny thing about the mix of blood and stool. The scent can linger on a surgeon's hands or feet for days, despite protective clothing. Its presence serves as a reminder of death left behind.

Almost immediately, the patient's blood pressure went to zero. His intestines were riddled with holes and he was exsanguinating from an injured iliac vein. It all literally fell apart between our hands. Within one minute, the man's heart stopped from shock and he went into cardiopulmonary arrest on the table. The efforts to resuscitate him were as futile as the attempt to operate and save him. He had been doomed as soon as the trigger was pulled. His death on the table, in our hands, had no meaning to me. He was just a case in my logbook, just a chance to operate. He was already dead before being rolled into the operating room.

During many years of practicing surgery in the community, I have often had to make decisions with life-and-death consequences, in complete cold-blooded isolation from any inner emotions or biases. Often, before I can even begin to process the consequences of these decisions, I am faced with another, and yet another. Some days, my job does not allow me the privilege of being human. Living at a distance from one's emotions can be a comfortable state to settle into. But despite the unique situations surgeons find themselves in daily, most are indeed very human. We may hide it well, but deep down our emotions percolate. Despite the urge to feel immortal after plucking out a ruptured spleen and saving a life, I am frequently reminded of my imperfections and mortality. My imperfections often arrive in the form of complications, such as accidentally making a hole in an artery or misdiagnosing a problem. My mortality often presents itself disguised as a patient.

Several years ago, I had the sad pleasure of operating on Mr. John Rogers. John was an active thirty-nine-year-old factory worker, with a wife, two young children, and the rest of his life ahead of him. When I opened him up in an attempt to remove his colon cancer, I discovered that the disease had already invaded many of his other organs. It was an extremely aggressive form of colon cancer. I did what I could, closed him up, and referred him for further treatment. He died six months later. Part of me saw myself in John, a healthy man going along in life until the divine plan abruptly comes to a halt. It was time to get a colonoscopy.

My biggest fear is bringing inadvertent harm to the patients I operate on, before, during, or after their operation. I live with this fear daily, even during the most mundane of operations. It doesn't consume me, but it is there. Surgery takes place on a fine line between benefit and harm. Although the fear of causing harm is still a constant, it was much worse when I started out in practice. When I was a new surgeon many years ago, my worst nightmare was the threat of a major complication or the unexpected death of a patient. I was fortunate to avoid the latter. It is often very difficult to recover, professionally and emotionally, from such disastrous outcomes early on in a surgical career.

One of my first operations in private practice was a laparoscopic cholecystectomy (removal of the gallbladder) on a woman with an acutely inflamed gallbladder. I thought the operation went well. I thought I had done all the correct things during the surgery. I had—except for one. Several days after the operation, the woman was having a lot of pain along with intermittent fever. I desperately wanted her course to go smoothly, not only for her sake but, frankly, for mine as well. I was partially blinded by my ego; I wanted my first patient to validate my self-worth by doing well. But I had missed the subtle signs. I should have carried out an x-ray procedure (called a cholangiogram) at the time of her operation. The cholangiogram would have prevented her complication. In the end, she had to undergo an additional procedure, additional pain, and a prolonged hospital stay. On my end, I needed to explain my thinking to the chief of surgery and required a prescription for the beginnings of an ulcer. The patient ultimately recovered. I aged five years for the five days she was in the hospital. I tried to disguise it, but I was an emotional mess taking care of her. I was my own surgeon now, responsible for my own complications. Residency had not prepared me for this very human moment. It was all new.

My biggest fear as a surgeon, a fear I often have to face, resurfaced one day in the form of a very pleasant grandmother of six. Several days before entering the hospital, Mrs. Grady had celebrated her seventy-fifth birthday. She had just finished a course of oral antibiotics to treat what her doctor described as a "touch of pneumonia" and was feeling good. With her three children and six grandchildren, she had enjoyed a lobster dinner at a local seafood restaurant. The place was famous for its three-and-a-half-pound baked lobsters stuffed with another pound of lobster meat. It was often difficult to finish off the giant beasts in one sitting. Mrs. Grady checked her cholesterol concerns at the door and dove in. Everyone had a great time and it wasn't until the next morning that she started having a little diarrhea. She did not think much of it as the day unfolded, thinking it might have been something she had eaten the night before. Toward evening, the diarrhea worsened and she started to feel weak. Then the cramping pains came. They were soon followed by fever. She was getting weaker and sicker and was on the verge of passing out. Her husband was panicking. He didn't know what was going on and brought her to the emergency room.

I had the pleasure of meeting Mrs. Grady at nine P.M. on a Tuesday night. Over the previous twenty-four hours this healthy, vibrant woman had been transformed into a dehydrated, critically ill patient with uncontrollable diarrhea. Her kidneys were also failing. Less than twenty-four hours ago, Mrs. Grady was enjoying chunks of lobster dipped in butter, surrounded by loved ones. Now she was slumped on an emergency room gurney, lethargic, experiencing waves of abdominal pain, and lying in her own diarrhea. The nurses could not keep up with her diaper pads. Mrs. Grady was going into septic shock from an evolving process inside her abdomen, a process caused by something given to millions of patients every day by their doctors across the country. A simple "touch of pneumonia" had brought Mrs. Grady to the brink of death and, coincidentally, to me, that night.

As a general surgeon, I am often called to evaluate patients with acute abdominal pain in the context of other symptoms. Many never need surgery because their complaints often resolve with medical treatment. Despite this, a select group of patients brings me to the darkest place in my mind. A select group that feeds on my biggest fear because of the diagnostic challenges they present. Once all the testing is done in this group, there are times I still haven't a clue what is going on inside their abdomen. In these patients, however, I am sure of one thing: Something deadly is evolving, deadly enough to require an operation to arrest it. In these cases, many patients undergo an exploratory laparotomy. The meaning of *exploratory* is self-evident. The word *laparotomy* originates from the Greek *lapara*, meaning to "cut." In the patient's world, it means I need to make a long cut through your abdominal wall, enter your abdominal cavity, and explore the organs inside. In my world, it means "I have no idea what the hell is happening in your abdomen and I need to get in there to find out or you die."

It is often as simple as that in many of these patients. Sure, I can sound official, button my long white coat, and reel off some names of different diagnoses. If this makes the patient's family feel more at ease, knowing that I have some idea what is going on, I am all too happy to do it. The bottom line is this: Patients in this critically ill group are in need of an emergent operation to stop the process unfolding inside their abdomen.

As I run through the mental checklist of why a patient may need an urgent exploratory laparotomy, I need to stop and dwell on one critical question. I need to ask myself, "Will the patient survive the operation?" Yes, you definitely need surgery as soon as possible, but will you wake up? This is a very important question to ask . . . and answer, if it can be answered at all. I need to use all my experience to come close to answering this question and presenting it honestly to the patient and family before any cut is made. I need to lay open the reality of the situation, delineate the expectations, and let the chips fall. There are times the answer is no, there is a good chance the patient will die; the stress of the illness, coupled with the trauma of surgery, will be too much. There are times when the answer is yes, there is a good chance the patient will survive the operation. And there are times when I have no idea whether a patient will survive surgery, with the caveat of a sure demise if nothing is done. To quote a famous colleague: "Surgery on the dying is often followed by death." Mrs. Grady was dying, and I did not want to hasten her death.

Her blood pressure was dropping, despite the heroic efforts of all the medical staff involved in her care. She was losing the battle raging inside her.

"Mr. Grady, how long was your wife on antibiotics?" I asked.

"About ten days." He could barely take his eyes off his wife. She was slipping into a coma.

"Nurse, has that stat *C. difficile* stool test come back?" I was pacing because I needed to make a decision now, a decision with life-and-death consequences. I was sure Mrs. Grady had contracted an infection in her large intestine (also called the colon) called *Clostridium difficile* colitis (also known as *C. diff* in medical jargon). She had contracted the infection from the oral antibiotics prescribed by her family physician. The antibiotics used to treat her pneumonia inadvertently wiped out some of the "good" bacteria living in her large intestine. These good bacteria are helpful in keeping other, more virulent bacteria, in check. Once removed, other dangerous bacteria (such as *C. difficile*), often dormant, come to life with a vengeance.

C. difficile colitis is fast becoming a major problem for patients in hospitals who are taking antibiotics for other reasons. It is becoming one of the more frequent hospital-acquired infections, leading to severe complications, surgery, and death. *C. difficile* actively infects the lining of the large intestine, causing profuse diarrhea, cramping, dehydration, renal failure, sepsis, and death if not treated appropriately. Ironically, the first line of treatment is another antibiotic, along with intravenous fluids. If medical treatment is not effective, the only other option is me, a general surgeon. My job here is to remove the offending organ, the large intestine, as quickly as possible. But putting someone through this type of major surgery is no guarantee that he or she will ever wake up. I am often called as a last resort, the cavalry, to make the final decision on life or death.

Part of me loves being in this position and part of me would like to crawl under a rock rather than face it. This is why I went into surgery, particularly general surgery. This is why I spent four fun years in college, two years working as an ironworker to save money, four years plugging away in medical school accumulating $100,000 in debt along the way, five years of learning how to operate, and three years fighting off insects the size of hamsters in the middle of the Louisiana Bayou serving my country. The moment had arrived. This is why my job is never boring. Among the elective, routine operations I often perform— repairing a hernia, removing a diseased gallbladder, taking out a thyroid gland—I *need* moments like this. Situations like this keep the fires burning deep inside the soul and never let me forget how human I am.

When I show up in these crisis situations, the family looks to me to be the savior, the one to stave off death and make their loved one whole. Part of me loves knowing that my physical skills give me the ability to make a difference *right now*. Something needs to be done, and I am the one to do it. Yet I am not pounding my own chest, not trumpeting my surgical skills, because moments like this also bring out the worst fear of all: the fear of being wrong when deciding to take a critically ill patient to the operating room. If I am wrong, my surgical skills, despite having the capability to save a life, can also take it away.

"Dr. Ruggieri, the *C. difficile* culture is positive."

I looked at Mrs. Grady's hopeless face while holding her trembling hand. I then glanced up at her husband. This was all I needed to know. The diagnosis was clear. In my mind the treatment was not. Often, patients with *C. difficile* colitis do improve with antibiotics and medical management. In some, the disease is self-limited, is cured with medicine, and doesn't progress to total organ failure and death. In others, the infection is relentless, does not respond to medical treatment, and progresses to death unless the offending organ (the large intestine) is removed. The key judgment I had to make was to decide when to operate and remove the infected large intestine during the course of the disease. If my decision is made too early in the disease process, I have put someone through the trauma of unnecessary surgery and left him or her with a permanent ileostomy. If my decision is made too late in the disease process, an operation will just be an exercise in futility, with death following. The timing has to be just right. Despite all the tests, the final decision to operate is a judgment call, similar to many of the urgent decisions most surgeons must make. The "art" of what I do is there for all to see. It is a decision made from current and past experiences, both good and bad. As I weighed the decision about Mrs. Grady, I had flashbacks of the faces of past patients in similar situations. There was Mr. Jacobson. He died soon after this type of surgery over a year ago. In retrospect, I might have waited too long on him. He was followed by Mrs. Berger, who still lives today. The decision to operate is made in complete isolation. It was nine thirty on a Tuesday night and the clock was ticking. This is why I wanted to be a surgeon. A decision had to made and acted on now.

I turned to Mr. Grady, "Sir, your wife is very sick and I have to decide whether to take her to the operating room now or wait twenty-four hours for medicine to work. If I wait too long to take her to the operating room, she will die. If I take her now, with the hope of stopping the infection, the stress of an operation could kill her." I was very blunt in my assessment. You have to be in these situations. You have to inform the family what they are up against. I was also naïvely searching for help in making my decision, foolishly thinking Mr. Grady might take some responsibility if I made the wrong decision and his wife did not make it. Was I looking to spread the accountability if Mrs. Grady did not make it off the operating room table? Who was I fooling? There was no one to help me now. I was alone.

"Doc, do whatever is necessary to save my wife." That was all he could muster.

Mrs. Grady had stopped making urine and her kidneys had completely shut down. It was time to go, time to get her to the operating room. It was time to be a surgeon.

Several weeks later, as I watched Mr. Grady help his recovering wife into their car for the drive home, I knew I had made the correct decision . . . this time. It felt good to be a surgeon today. Why did she live and Mr. Jacobson, my patient from a year ago, die? What was different here? My hesitation? Was it just luck? As the car pulled away from the hospital entrance, I thanked the patients that had come before Mrs. Grady, thanked them for helping me make the right decision to operate. Many of the urgent life-and-death decisions I make as a surgeon are based on lessons learned from "bad" experiences. The sad truth is this: Some people get hurt (or even die) as surgeons develop their skills. I have learned a great deal from the patients I have helped—and from those I have hurt. Mrs. Grady's experience was extremely rewarding on many levels. I relished the moment, closing my eyes and allowing the warmth of the sun to lick my face. Unfortunately, summer's end came quickly as my pager started to go off.

"Dr. Ruggieri, please call the emergency room."

///

In addition to living with the emotional consequences of life-and-death decisions, I (as well as many of my colleagues) am often looked upon by patients as having all the answers. Frequently, I am viewed as the all-knowing surgeon, the person with the power to diagnose an illness and cure it with an operation. Patients tend to view surgeons as Godlike, possessing the skills to help them live another day. I am supposed to be perfect every moment of every single day. Believe me, I desperately want to be perfect in every decision I make, outside or inside the operating room. I was trained to expect nothing less than perfection and groomed to be perfect by society's expectations. I wish I had all the answers to every patient's illness, but I do not. It has taken time to live comfortably with my human imperfections and limitations. On most days, with most patients, I have the correct answers (otherwise I would not have a practice). There are surgeons who are unable to accept their imperfections, to learn from their humility. Some are unable to admit that they do not know everything, unable to face failure and accept blame. Some of them can hide their human flaws well behind the closed doors of an operating room.

As a surgeon in practice, I consider myself as human as any other working person. On a professional level, I know I am a highly trained "technician" whose workplace is unique. My professional successes and failures result in human consequences, often visible for all to observe. If a stockbroker has a bad day picking stocks, his 401(k) and retirement accounts suffer in silence. If I have a bad day in my workplace, people suffer. If a stockbroker has a stellar day of trading, his clients are financially better off for it. If I have a stellar day in the operating room (every day should be stellar), my clients are physically better off for it. In many ways, surgeons are no different professionally or personally from a stockbroker, an engineer, or a plumber. We all have in common specific job insecurities; experience good, bad, and better days; lose patience on occasion, don't feel like getting up some mornings, wish we could make more money, often do not realize what we have, and sometimes don't say what we truly mean.

For me, one of my deepest job insecurities, outside my fear of inadvertently harming patients by my decisions or actions, revolves around my reputation as general surgeon in the community. Like any laborer in the public workforce, I take enormous pride in my work and allow it to speak for itself. As a surgeon in private practice, I rely on my reputation to sustain my business. It is who I am and validates my self-worth as a human being. The worth of my abilities shapes how I define myself in society. Surgeons' good reputations are built over time, through a combination of hard work, competent decisions, compassion, and, most important, good patient outcomes. Without good patient outcomes, it does not matter how nice a person you may be. If most of my patients do not do well after surgery, my practice will suffer, as well it should. Ultimately, every operation I perform is a testimonial.

Most of the patients I have chosen to operate on do well. The key word here is *chosen*. The patients who have suffered complications, or have not made it through surgery, are the ones who lead me to another insecurity: the fear of being sued. This fear is real for all doctors, but especially so for surgeons. In today's simmering legal climate, some surgeons view every patient they take to the operating room as a potential lawsuit. When a patient has a bad outcome, the first thing on my mind is the safety of the patient and what I can do to correct the bad outcome. The second thing? A lawsuit. Bad outcomes equal potential lawsuits. Surgeons have to be able to look past this fear or their practices become hobbled by time and money wasted on unnecessary tests. Studies show that the risk of getting sued is small and, when it does occur, most doctors are exonerated in the end. Recent studies have also shown that doctors may overexaggerate this fear in their heads. There are surgeons who worry that every patient is a potential lawsuit and others who never give it a thought. I fall somewhere in between.

Surgeons, like many professionals, have other job insecurities. We worry about the source of future referrals—future income—to pay future personal expenses. Doctors, in general, often worry needlessly about money, and surgeons are a special breed of worrier. Surgeons are a special breed because of the lifestyle they are able to lead, a lifestyle that costs money. I am a specialist and I make money by performing operations. My business is based on referrals. Without referrals from other doctors (internists, gastroenterologists, and so on), I do not have a practice. Without a practice, I cannot pay my mortgage or college tuition. In today's market, whether I like it or not, I have to be vigilant in monitoring the shifting local politics of medicine in order to stay competitive. In private practice, physician practices are constantly being bought out by bigger groups or hospitals, sometimes forcing a change in referral patterns. Today, referrals to specialists are no longer based solely on the quality of care a specialist provides. In an ideal world, good surgeons would be referred business regardless of which group they belong to or align themselves with. I do not practice in an ideal world.

As a member of the human race, I frequently experience an array of emotions, urges, and thoughts throughout the workweek on which I may or may not act. Most of the time, I can disguise or compartmentalize them well enough to function at a very high level. At other times, my human side gets the best of me. My profession as a surgeon does not exempt me from acting like a normal person when angry, sad, happy, or disgusted. There have been times when I have been angry at patients because of their behavior. When I caught a patient trying to steal needles and syringes from my office, I threw him out. There have been times when I have been upset with myself for making stupid decisions, such as accidentally cutting across an artery during an operation because I was in a hurry to finish a case. There have been times when I have refused to operate on people electively (not emergently) because I determined that an operation, given their poor medical health, would kill them. I have also refused to operate on patients because I believed their symptoms would not improve despite what the tests (and even other surgeons) might indicate. I have had the pleasure of experiencing the extremes of human emotions, thanks to my work. Mr. Richmond was one such case.

In a span of eight hours, a patient I will call Mr. Harold Richmond took me from the emotional high of knowing I had performed the most complex thyroid cancer surgery perfectly to the low of the most scared-shitless fifteen minutes of my life. Six hours after his thyroidectomy for cancer, Mr. Richmond started to bleed into his neck. A blood vessel had broken loose. A patient can bleed suddenly after surgery when a tie placed during the operation around a blood vessel comes undone (most likely because it was not secured properly in the first place). A patient can also bleed because of carelessness on the surgeon's part, or from plain bad luck. An operative field can look bone-dry at the time I close the skin, yet the chance exists that I'll get a call in the middle of the night.

Mr. Richmond was bleeding into his neck. If something wasn't done soon, he would suffocate from his own blood. Jamie, the astute nurse taking care of him, alerted me to his deteriorating condition.

"Mr. Richmond, are you getting enough air?" He winced but nodded. His expanding neck was blowing up like a balloon. I knew I didn't have much time to get him back to the O.R. His airway was being compressed from the blood clots. He was suffocating. I had to reopen his neck and evacuate the blood.

The ride down the elevator to the operating room was the longest ten seconds of my life. As the doors closed, all I could think of was him going into respiratory arrest in the elevator, dying between the third and second floor. I had to get to the O.R.

This is not going to be good, I thought. *This man is going from being the most textbook of thyroid operations to dying in an elevator on the way to the first floor. How am I going to live with this death on my hands? What am I going to tell the family?* All I could do was force a smile as I watched twenty-five years of school, training, and practice fade away as Mr. Richmond continued to bleed. It would be difficult, emotionally and professionally, to recover from this one.

My practice is over. It's over. Forget the college tuition, forget the vacations. See you in court. Time to find another job. The elevator doors opened and I snapped back to reality. I looked down at Mr. Richmond's face. It had a mild blue hue to it, but he was still breathing.

"Mr. Richmond, stay with me." He nodded. He wasn't dead yet. There was still a chance. The operating room was ready, and we shoved him on the table as fast as we could. I quickly splashed his neck with antiseptic solution and slit his neck incision wide open. The blood clots burst out of his neck as the anesthesiologist was placing a breathing tube in his trachea. All those years of training were not wasted after all, or so I thought.

"Is the breathing tube in?" I searched for the anesthesiologist's eyes. My hands were shaking. "What the hell is going on up there?" I could barely see over the drapes.

"Cannot get the breathing tube in. There is just too much swelling." The sweat was visible on the anesthesiologist's face.

"Shit. Get me a tracheotomy set and number six trach now." I could barely contain my shaking. My left leg started to twitch. Mr. Richmond's face was turning a darker blue from lack of oxygen. I had to trach the guy now or he would be brain dead. There was no room for error. This was the moment of truth, the fine line between life and death that exists in my workplace. It was either put the tracheostomy tube in now or call the funeral home. I had created this moment, and I needed to finish it.

At the end of the surgery, Mr. Richmond was awake, alert, and getting plenty of oxygen from a newly placed tracheostomy tube. Everything was moving. His brain function was intact. He would survive. Six hours earlier, I was on top of the world after a perfect thyroid operation. Now I was completely drained, exhausted from this brush with death. As I watched the operating nurses change his blood-soaked gown, I felt something warm between my legs. I looked down and could only smile, realizing I needed a change of underwear before going to my office.

///

Are surgeons truly human? How does your surgeon block out all the negative noise, all the pressures of the job, and keep it tightly together on the day of your hip replacement, hysterectomy, hernia operation, or heart bypass surgery? On the day of your surgery, would you even know it if your surgeon had been up all night, was going through a bitter divorce, or had lost a patient an hour earlier?

The truth is that surgeons are *very* human, perhaps only appearing to behave in superhuman ways despite personal and professional adversity. There are days when I do not want to see or listen to *any* patients. There are days when the compassion in me has been nearly drained out by fatigue or stress. I have days when I second-guess the decisions I have made both inside and outside the operating room. Days when the last thing I want to do is to explain to a patient's family that their loved one's cancer has spread and I could not remove it all. On the other hand, I also have days when I surprise myself with all the correct decisions that were made, all the perfect work that was done, carried out in the unpredictable, high-stakes world of the operating room.

Despite human frailties and weaknesses, most of the surgeons I know are ordinary people who can do extraordinary things. They are focused individuals who, despite personal or professional adversity, are capable of helping patients and saving lives. I have had the privilege of knowing surgeons of all shapes, sizes, skills, and personalities—honest and dishonest, including egomaniacs who think they are gods, think they can do no wrong and lay blame on everyone but themselves. These are the ones who lay the blame on nurses or "faulty" instruments for their mishaps in the operating room. Some of them couldn't operate their way out of a paper bag. Then there are those whose skills I can only envision in my dreams. I have operated with surgeons whose humility is as sharp as their surgical skills—these are the best of my breed, the ones who stay humble. I have seen surgeons cry with families, sharing in the grief of the unexpected loss of a loved one. I have also observed surgeons who care only about themselves and the almighty dollar. Most of the surgeons I know, the ones with whom I am honored to count myself as a colleague, are dedicated, intelligent, compassionate individuals who put a patient's welfare above all else. It's what we've been trained to do.

Chapter 3

First, Try Not to Harm

Every day, my head throbbed before entering his room. I was afraid, angry, and partly in denial at what I had created. I had been given one chance with this frail man, one try to get him through the trauma of a major operation without complications. A chance I'd blown. Despite the fear and anger, I had no choice but to face the situation. He was my patient, my responsibility. I could not pawn him off on another surgeon in another city. I had to see him through this ordeal. I had to fix the problem I'd created during his surgery.

Ten days earlier, I had purposely invaded his abdominal cavity to remove a cancerous growth in his colon. I thought the operation went well; it seemed to meet my expectations. Later, I would learn how wrong I was.

As I approached the door to his hospital room, sweat was making its way through my shirt. Today, I had on my long white coat. I needed it. I needed its security, its symbolic armor to help get me through my visit with Mr. Andrews. I often put it on when I want to look official before entering a tense, potentially hostile situation. I paused at the doorway, just beyond the sight of Mrs. Andrews, mentally rehearsing what I wanted to say about her husband's condition, the cause of this unexpected "complication." I needed to choose my words carefully. The wrong words, spoken at an inappropriate time to patients and their families, can come back to haunt you. Surgeons (if you can pin them down long enough to get an answer) like to speak in generalities about complications, without getting specific about the root cause. The reason: Most patients *do* recover from their complications, alleviating the need for surgeons to ever approach discussing anything like an explanation. With Mr. Andrews, I had to walk a fine line, offering enough hope about his recovery without being unrealistic.

I stood there, motionless, for what seemed like an eternity, fending off the ghosts of my past complications. Every new surgical complication brings back memories of past imperfections, along with the guilt, humiliation, and lessons learned from each one. Most of my patients do well. The sad truth, though, is that many of them have no lasting memory in my mind. There are just too many faces to remember, too many gallbladders removed, too many hernias repaired. These faces get replaced by others as time goes by. For the small minority who have experienced poor outcomes (including death) over the course of my career, the guilt and remorse resurface with each new complication.

I can also vividly remember the first, and only, patient who died on the operating room table under my knife early on in private practice. He had a perforated stomach ulcer. By the time I decided to take him to the operating room, sepsis (infection) had set in from a hole in his stomach leaking gastric juices. The trauma of an operation was the last nail in the coffin. In retrospect, the surgery had been an exercise in futility. He went into cardiopulmonary arrest on the table after I opened him up, never making it out of the operating room. I wept with the family in the waiting room after informing them of the outcome. I wept for their loss. I could not save him. Could I have intervened sooner? Again, the lessons of past experiences are vital for determining when to intervene to prevent harm or death. I was slowly beginning to learn them, along with the high emotional cost.

Despite the lessons of imperfection learned from experiences and despite my security as a "reputable" surgeon, I was very apprehensive standing outside Mr. Andrews's room. I dreaded having to face his nervous wife, her sad eyes desperately seeking good news. All she wanted to hear was that her husband was improving and would be all right. That is all most patients and their families want to hear when things go wrong. I could not, honestly, tell her what she wanted to hear. Most of all, I dreaded facing my shame, my surgical mistake lying there exposed for all to see.

Mr. Andrews was referred to me because a cancerous tumor had been found in his cecum, the first portion of his large intestine. He had seen his primary care doctor for an annual checkup. The man felt fine, no complaints, no pain, eating well. As all doctors do, his had ordered blood tests even though this was a "routine" visit. (Patients cannot escape a doctor's office without getting stuck with a needle for blood tests. Most blood tests are explained to patients as "routine." Patients are also informed that they will hear from the doctor's office "in a few days" if anything abnormal is discovered. A few days can turn into a few weeks, and a few weeks into no news at all. Never assume that no news is good news; the test results may have been misplaced or lost.) Unfortunately, the results were far from routine for Mr. Andrews. His hemoglobin, a measure of his red blood cell count, was low.

He was shocked to be seeing a surgeon, and apprehensive of hearing the C-word. "But, Doc, I have never had any pain." For most cancers, pain doesn't show up as a symptom until the disease has spread to the rest of the body. Once over the shock of hearing the word *cancer*, patients are perplexed, particularly when there were never any noticeable symptoms.

Mr. Andrews continued to focus on the fact that he had no pain. I listened as he wondered out loud how this could have happened, while I thought about the operation in his future. His red blood cell count was low enough to establish a warning sign in his doctor's mind. A low hemoglobin in an otherwise apparently healthy patient in his age group—seventies and eighties— is cancer of the gastrointestinal tract until proven otherwise. I would never say this before further testing confirmed it. There are many thoughts I would never share with patients upon first meeting them. There are some things patients just do not need to know before (or after) their operation, especially if complications arise. In the case of Mr. Andrews, his problem and the solution would soon be very clear.

There are patients with illnesses (cancer is not one of them) who fall into a large "gray zone," patients with illnesses that may not improve with an operation. Surgeons have to choose their patients wisely in order to maximize the opportunity for a good result. I tend to be more conservative when recommending surgery if, in my mind, things are not clear-cut. Over my career, I have lost some business because of this and pissed off some referring doctors in the process. There are surgeons (and I know some of them) who will operate on anyone with a pulse, despite the lack of strong evidence supporting a good outcome. This type of surgeon is motivated by greed, ego, or insecurity. When unsuspecting patients cross paths with such a surgeon, harm can result.

///

In my practice as a general surgeon, by the time I see you in my office, something needs to be either removed, repaired, or biopsied. This is what I do. I do not exist to talk about your heartburn, neck pain, weight gain, fatigue, or swollen legs. This is not my job and, frankly, I'm not interested. You have a specific surgical problem and I have a specific answer: an operation. I chose surgery as a medical specialty because I like to work with and rely on my hands; this is how I want to improve your health. I want my *surgical skills*—not some medication—to be responsible in healing your illness. When I examine a patient, my mind is always engaged in the same puzzle, trying to decide (based on symptoms and test results) if the person before me needs (and will benefit from) surgery. If I decide you will, I need to make sure you understand what the most realistic expectations of outcome are—including what can go wrong. This is one of the first places for surgeons to do harm to patients, by misjudging the situation and operating on someone for the wrong reasons. Some surgeons, even before they place a knife on you, have caused you harm by recommending surgery. This is one of the first stops in the patient-surgeon relationship that can be hazardous to your health.

My approach, once I have finalized my decision, is to be frank with patients. As for Mr. Andrews, a routine checkup leads to discovering a low blood count, which leads to a colonoscopy, which leads to the discovery of colon cancer, which leads (finally) to a visit with me. "Mr. and Mrs. Andrews, it is a pleasure to meet you both. I need to take out several feet of your colon, sir. Does next week sound good?" How life can change with a routine trip to your primary care physician's office.

As Mr. Andrews and his wife sat in my office describing the events that led up to his visit with me, only part of me was listening. Have you ever wondered to what extent your doctor actually *listens* to your complaints during the office visit? For surgeons, strategic listening is crucial in deciding, particularly for certain conditions, whether an operation will be of benefit. There are times I find myself not listening to a patient's entire story, but rather filtering through the fluff to understand the meat of the symptoms. Unfortunately, my listening abilities have diminished exponentially with the passing of time, only to be surpassed by the decline in my ability to write legibly.

With Mr. Andrews, I was already focusing on his upcoming operation. *The man has a colon cancer. It needs to come out.* With this knowledge, I have initiated the subconscious process of "sizing him up" medically. *What is his risk of a complication or death? How difficult is this operation going to be for me based on his body shape and weight? Has he had previous abdominal surgery? Has another surgeon been in his abdomen already, creating scar tissue I will now have to deal with?* I often cringe when I find a long abdominal scar on a patient I need to operate on. Previous surgery creates scar tissue, which in turn makes my job inside and outside the operating room more difficult. In addition to increasing the risk of "collateral" damage inside the operating room, previous surgery can lead to a prolonged recovery time in the hospital. *What are Mr. Andrews's chances of surviving if the operation does not go perfectly?* He is a frail, eighty-one-year-old man with underlying chronic medical conditions, conditions that put him, or anyone like him, at risk for complications.

Most elderly patients who come to me for major abdominal surgery fit into this category. People are living longer, developing cancer at a later age, and often undergoing major surgery. It is well documented that older people are at a higher risk for complications and death after any major operation. The older you are, the higher the risk. As a surgeon, I can often surmise how well a patient will do before even entering the operating room. In addition to age, other surgical risk factors in patients increase the risk for complications after surgery. These include obesity, diabetes, history of smoking, and heart disease. I swallow hard when I have to schedule an obese patient, with diabetes (or other chronic illnesses), who smokes, for major abdominal surgery, knowing full well things may not go perfectly. This type of patient, today the norm and not the exception, is a setup for life-threatening complications. And many older patients are returning with new surgical problems resulting from a previous operation.

I would love to turn these high-risk patients away at the door, happy to find them another surgeon. This is not as easy as it sounds. I make my living operating, and I need to be smart in deciding whom to take to the operating room. There are times, because of lack of experience, that I may not want to operate on a patient. I may decline because I believe the operation is too much for me to handle. There are also times when I know an outcome is not going to be perfect, and I do not want to be the one responsible for it. I will bluntly let patients know this; I want them to understand that it is in their best interest for me not to operate. Here, my ego will gladly step aside and allow the reality of daily practice to take over. I can absorb only so many major mistakes, so many bad outcomes or deaths before my work invites close scrutiny, my reputation gets blackened, and my referrals dry up. Even in the practice of surgery, there is a Darwinian natural selection process, a survival of the fittest.

Inside and outside the hospital, surgeons are being watched very closely today. In today's healthcare environment, complications after surgery raise red flags within hospital quality-control departments. Whenever a major complication arises after an operation, the quality-control folks (both administrators and physicians) stand ready to document, investigate, and pass judgment. Doctors today, especially surgeons, are living in the ever-expanding world of Big Brother.

Toward the end of my explanation of how I would remove about two feet of Mr. Andrews's colon and reconnect his small and large intestine, I could sense both husband and wife sizing me up. I could see by the expressions on their faces that they were trying to decide if I was competent and experienced enough (meaning old enough) to perform the operation. This is the million-dollar question when you are sitting across the desk from a surgeon. Sure, all of us have the necessary diplomas, training, and board certification credentials on our walls, proving to the world how competent we are. Yes, we have performed enough surgery to be considered competent to practice by the state licensing boards. Despite this, the question every patient asks himself is the same: *Is my surgeon competent enough to perform my surgery safely? Will he or she be in top form on the day of my operation? Has he or she done enough of these operations?* All good questions, but what they probably are not asking (and should) is, *Can this surgeon get out of trouble in the operating room, trouble he or she created?* Good surgeons know how to get themselves out of their own trouble in the operating room and deal with unexpected, or self-made, complications. How do you, as a patient, know this? This information does not appear, framed, hanging on a wall in my office. My complication rates do not appear on a certificate. The mortality rates for the operations I perform are not printed on a chart for your review.

Ultimately, I took Mr. Andrews to the operating room and removed about a foot of his right colon for a cancerous tumor.

The cancer had not spread to other organs and he was essentially cured with surgery. The operation went well. At least, that was what I believed at the time. He was discharged in seven days after an uneventful hospital course and with minimal pain. I was ecstatic to see him leave without something bad happening. He was old and frail, and the operation had taken a lot out of him. At the time of discharge, the patient was happy because he had done well and been discharged without complications. The patient's wife was happy because the cancer had not spread and had been safely removed. The referring internist was happy because Mr. Andrews did well and that made him look good in referring him to me. I was happy because everything appeared to have gone according to plan.

Before entering his room, I took a deep breath, rehearsed my words, and put my best surgeon face on. It was exhausting to face Mr. Andrews and his wife, trying to convince her on a daily basis that the "complication" resulting from her husband's colon surgery would eventually heal. It was an emotionally exhausting effort to keep her confident in her husband's full recovery. Her eyes could only see a vigorous husband of fifty-one years losing weight and hope daily. "His condition remains stable and he is not losing any ground. I just do not know when he will be able to eat solid food. Let's see how he looks tomorrow." My right eyelid started to twitch uncontrollably, a reaction I have experienced for years as a result of prolonged fatigue, stress, and too much coffee. (It freaked me out the first time it occurred. It happened on one long night during training. I was in the middle of learning how to perform an appendectomy. The suddenness of onset almost caused me to accidentally plunge a scalpel into my left thumb.) I struggled to maintain direct eye contact with both Mr. and Mrs. Andrews. I could offer nothing more at this point, wanting desperately to get out of there.

Mr. Andrews had returned to the hospital ten days after his colon cancer surgery. I met him and his wife in the emergency room. No surgeon is happy to get a call from the emergency room about a recently operated-on patient. A call like this gets me thinking about the worst-case scenario. It also erases all the personal and professional satisfaction already processed on Mr. Andrews at the time of his uncomplicated discharge. "Doctor, my husband was doing so well from his surgery until yesterday." I did not utter a word. She pointed to the green-stained bandage covering his incision. I knew right away, by the color, by the foul odor of the fluid underneath, what I was dealing with. I did not want to remove the bandage, did not want to come face-to-face with my imperfection.

I pulled back the dressing. A foul-smelling greenish fluid slowly percolated up from a dark opening in his abdominal incision. Mrs. Andrews's eyes widened with disbelief. I felt nauseated. She was horrified by the sight of the problem. I was nauseated because of what the next few weeks in the hospital would bring for him and me. I was already racing ahead, envisioning the upcoming legal depositions, the questions to answer, and the ultimate price to be paid if he did not get over this. I paused for a moment, carefully selecting my next words. "I am sorry, sir, but you have a serious problem related to the surgery and need to be admitted into the hospital." That was all I could muster for now without being pressed for answers. I was hoping none would be required just yet. I was not ready to throw open the truth gates. "Was it something I did?" Mr. Andrews was looking for answers while I was looking for a rock to crawl under. I would have loved to answer yes. I would have loved to shift the burden of blame away from me and rationalize my mistake by blaming someone or something else. I could not do it.

Mr. Andrews had developed an enterocutaneous fistula, a connection between his small intestine and the skin. This is a serious complication that can occur after intestinal surgery, especially in someone who is already in a weakened state. It often requires a prolonged and costly hospitalization, intravenous feedings, antibiotics, and, sometimes, further surgery to close the connection. Patients cannot eat for weeks, in order to give the connection time to seal itself off. All of this is stressful for the patient, family, and operating surgeon. Can it happen? Of course. Does it happen? Yes. I just never wanted it to happen to me. In Mr. Andrews's case, the connection between his small intestine and large intestine, the connection I created, had leaked bacteria-laden juices sometime after the surgery. While leaking, intestinal juices follow the path of least resistance to the skin. This is considered a technical complication of the operation. It is technical in the sense that my operative technique failed to create an airtight connection after his cancer removal. As much as I was searching for a scapegoat, there was no one to blame but myself. This one was on my surgical watch. I had no choice but to deal with it.

All Mr. Andrews wanted was a piece of toast or some juice.

Something cold, something liquid to moisten the cracks on his lips. Unfortunately, I could not allow it. It would worsen his condition, provide false gratification, and prolong his hospitalization. My heart ached to feed him. Here I was, the cause of this complication, adding insult to injury by denying him food. I wanted to show his wife he was making some progress by a simple gesture, a glass of juice. An offer of a beverage would have restored some of her confidence in me. But it was too early in the process and I could not allow it. I desperately wanted his body to recover from this insult, wanted him to leave the hospital as soon as possible. I wanted to hasten his recovery and get him out of the hospital before more bad things happened.

Hospitals can be dangerous places, despite the medical miracles often performed in them. Close to 100,000 patients die each year in American hospitals from infections acquired while they are patients, and this number is rising despite all the improvements and money injected into our hospital systems ever since the Institute of Medicine published a landmark study in 1999 that shocked the entire country. This sentinel report revealed that anywhere from 44,000 to 98,000 patients die in hospitals every year from "medical errors," many of which involve unnecessary infections. Yes, I was extremely anxious to get Mr. Andrews out of the hospital because with every passing day, his risk of getting a hospital-acquired infection increased. In someone who is already compromised from the trauma of a surgical complication, a blood infection would be a death knell. It would be the final insult, stacked on top of what I had already given him. I did not want this on my watch. I had to do whatever I could to stay on top of his progress and prevent his condition from deteriorating past the physiological point of no return.

I also wanted Mr. Andrews out of the hospital as soon as possible for selfish reasons. I wanted the guilt to go away. I wanted to close the door on this one and not be reminded of my imperfection every single day. I wanted him out so I could stop torturing myself in bed with the *why*s and *what if*s. I wanted to sleep at night. I wanted to shut the multitude of eyes keenly monitoring how all patients do after surgery. These eyes are attached to hands, hands that are tabulating monthly complication rates, taking notes, and handing out performance report cards at the end of each quarter. Most of all, I did not want Mr. Andrews to die in the hospital, to die because of a mistake in judgment I made at the time of his surgery. This is every surgeon's nightmare, a nightmare that will be revisited in front of colleagues at monthly department meetings, sometimes resurrected later in a court of law, and never forgotten.

As the next day turned into the next week, I knew Mr. Andrews would be in for a prolonged hospital course. I grappled with how to explain to him the nature of his complication. Several studies have shown that when faced with bad outcomes, surgeons are cautious in discussing the real cause. It is difficult for me to use the word *mistake* or *error* in any explanation. The power of a surgeon's words is considerably magnified in the setting of a surgical complication. With each passing day without food, each pound lost, I could feel the Andrewses' hope and confidence in me dying. With each passing day, a part of me was dying as well.

Complications, surgical errors, and poor outcomes have been and will continue to be an unfortunate, often unspoken, aspect of my profession. This is nothing new to surgeons who practice surgery on a daily basis. Unnecessary harm and unexpected death can happen to anyone after any operation by any surgeon. There is no discrimination by gender, race, or social class. It's a daily fact: Not every operation goes perfectly, and not every patient leaves the hospital with a good outcome. My profession, like many other aspects of medicine, is not an exact science. There are too many variables at play from the minute a patient steps into a surgeon's office until the time he or she leaves the hospital. One of these variables is that your surgeon is human, trying to obtain perfection in a complex, imperfect world. I am not programmed with the ability to have perfect hand technique and judgment in the operating room every day. I wish I were. I did know a surgeon during training who came very close to being the perfect operating machine. He was a heart surgeon (I will call him Dr. G), king of the surgical totem pole. The man had hands of gold with operating skills second only to a divine being. He made the most complex heart surgery look effortless. His God-given talents often gave his patients the best chance for a good outcome. He was the best of the best. He knew it and so did everyone else. He was the closest thing to a perfect technician inside the operating room that I had ever seen. Despite the physical talent, he did not have the warmest of bedside manners. He did not have it all. None of us ever do.

There are adverse events—things that happen beyond a surgeon's control—that can ruin the most perfect of operations. One of Dr. G's most high-profile patients, the father of a prominent cardiologist, suffered a massive stroke after his heart bypass surgery and never woke up. It was a devastating event for all involved and totally unrelated to the operating skills of Dr. G that day. The stroke was one of those variables that can affect a surgical patient, regardless of the skill of the surgeon. Yes, the operation went well, but the patient never left the hospital.

I wish I could be perfect inside the operating room every day. I wish every one of my patients would do as well as I think he or she should. I wish I would never unintentionally harm another patient again. Unfortunately, I know my wishes will never all come true.

As a general surgeon, I mainly operate on organs in the neck and inside the abdomen. I can perform surgery on a variety of organs, such as the intestine, gallbladder, and thyroid gland, for a variety of reasons. When you are in practice long enough, mistakes in surgical technique and judgment will find you. I have run the gamut on all the major complications, inside and outside the operating room, specific to the operations I perform. You name it, I (and most active surgeons today) have experienced it. I have cut into major blood vessels by accident, inadvertently made holes in the intestine during surgery, accidentally cut the main bile duct off the gallbladder, inadequately connected two pieces of intestine (Mr. Andrews comes to mind), and mistakenly damaged the nerve controlling the vocal cords during thyroid surgery. I am not proud of these complications and would love to take every one of them, and the suffering attached, back. Every active surgeon has experienced errors in judgment inside and outside the operating room, errors that have harmed patients. These human errors can occur during the simplest of operations or the most complex. They do not discriminate. We all have skeletons in our professional closet (some surgeons have bigger closets than others), skeletons we deal with on a daily basis. At the end of the day, all I can do is the best I can.

How common are surgical complications? Recent studies indicate that up to 13 percent of general/vascular surgery patients in private hospitals experience a complication after an operation. Of these patients, close to 2 percent never make it out of the hospital. Is the existence of mistakes and complications new in surgery? No. Are they increasing in number? I doubt it. The record keeping and public sharing of data is what's new and, I believe, accounts for the growing numbers. Today, external forces, both financial and quality improvement related, are reshaping the culture of silence that has existed in the surgical profession for years.

Surgeons have the potential to make an error in judgment while caring for you. The potential exists from the minute you walk into the office to the time you are discharged from the hospital. Even the most routine of operations has the potential to be imperfect at any point along the process. Every single decision I make that will affect a patient before or after an operation has its own unique set of consequences. In addition, the many judgments I make inside the operating room have the potential to adversely affect your outcome. The wrong judgments inside the operating room are the ones with the most influence on your postoperative course. Mistakes made inside the operating room by surgeons come in all shapes and sizes. Most of these mistakes, when they occur, will have been immediately recognized by your surgeon and corrected before you leave the operating room. This is one of the qualities of a good surgeon: the ability to recognize and correct the unexpected error made inside the operating room. The errors that go unrecognized at the time of an operation are the ones that cause the most harm to patients. Some lead to a second operation; others can lead to death.

The most tragic of these in my specialty is the unsuspected hole made in the intestine at the time of an operation. Laparoscopic surgery is commonplace today and performed for a variety of diseases inside the abdominal cavity. Its enormous benefits to patients are well documented, starting with a faster recovery. But the benefits can come with a cost. Laparoscopic removal of the gallbladder is one of the most common operations I do. During this type of operation, sharp devices are inserted blindly into the abdominal cavity to facilitate the surgery. Most of the time, these devices enter safely. They have the potential, however, to perforate the intestine. If this injury goes unrecognized, it can lead to significant morbidity. Does it happen often? Not at all. Can it happen? Yes. The entire country was introduced to this complication with the death of a well-known congressman from Pennsylvania after he underwent "routine" laparoscopic gallbladder surgery at a prominent teaching hospital.

Fortunately, most of the recognized errors corrected inside the operating room will never influence your outcome. You will also never know about them. Some errors will lead to further surgery, and some may even inadvertently kill you. With Mr. Andrews, I was convinced the connection I made at the time of his operation was sound. I believed it because I thought I did everything correctly, as I had done hundreds of times before.

A recent study from a major Boston teaching program reviewed all incidents causing disability and death in surgical patients. This study revealed that two-thirds of these incidents involved a surgical error during an operation. Of these, 66 percent involved a technical error, meaning a problem created during the actual operation, and 33 percent involved an error in judgment. The technical error I made during Mr. Andrews's operation was an inadequate connection between his small and large intestine after the cancer was removed. Studies have tried to shed light on why mistakes occur by asking surgeons themselves. One such study revealed burnout as a significant contributor to the cause of surgical errors. In this study, 9 percent of surgeons (out of close to eight thousand asked) stated they had made a major medical error in the last three months. This does not surprise me. Other factors that have been shown to contribute to problems inside the operating room and subsequent poor outcomes include experience and judgment (closely linked), inadequate physical skills, fatigue, carelessness, rushing, ego and incompetence (also closely linked), and, believe it or not, the patient.

Experience and proper judgment are two of the most important safeguards against errors in the operating room. Every surgeon possesses a unique set of experiences (which include mistakes made and solutions rendered), based on his or her training and practice history. These experiences are filed away in our memory library, called upon as a guide to help us make the safe and correct judgment when things get stressful. During the early years of my practice, I was continually honing my skills. Yes, I was licensed to practice, had all the credentials, and was a "safe" surgeon. But I was also gaining vital experience and skill with each operation. When I made a mistake, I learned how to correct it.

During the second ten years of my practice, I continued to learn the lesson of *when* to operate. One of the key factors for staying out of trouble in the operating room is choosing the right patient for the right reasons. In Mr. Andrews's case, he was the correct patient to operate on and for the correct reasons.

How do you, as a patient, know when the surgeon in front of you has enough experience to give you the best chance for a successful operation? Studies have shown what most of us know intuitively: Inside the operating room, practice makes perfect. Do not be afraid to ask your surgeon how many operations he or she has performed. Does this guarantee success? Of course not. Do not be afraid to ask your surgeon to explain the potential major complications specific to your operation. Ask, "What is the normal major complication rate for my operation? What is your complication rate for my operation?" The answers should come quickly. And if the answer to the last question is zero, I would be polite, leave, and find another surgeon. Do not be afraid to ask your surgeon how he or she manages complications specific to your operation. For instance, I perform a lot of thyroid surgery in my practice, and the main complication is damage to the nerves controlling the voice, leaving it weak and hoarse. A very few times (quite rarely, as a matter of fact, otherwise I would not be doing thyroid surgery), I have damaged this nerve during surgery, permanently affecting the voice of a patient. I tell prospective patients about this during the consultation, including how often it has happened and how to correct it. Initially, it shocks them that I will admit this. Most of them listen, respect my honesty, and allow me to do their surgery.

I must admit, fatigue and impatience have undoubtedly contributed to some mistakes I have made in the operating room. Some abdominal operations can last for five, six, or even seven hours, depending on the problem. Because I am human, I get tired, especially if the surgery is taking place in the middle of the night. Most surgeons are used to operating, and operating well, in a fatigued state. It is something we learn during training and carry with us as a badge of honor. As far as the impatience goes, ask any operating room nurse and you will hear that surgeons are "always in a hurry." They are in a hurry to get you out of their office. They are in a hurry to see you in the morning, and in a hurry to leave after your operation. They are in a hurry to get into the operating room, and once there, they are in a hurry to get out. Surgeons are also in a hurry to get you out of the hospital after surgery. This impatience, I believe, originates from the days of surgical training. Surgical residents have so much work to do in a twenty-four-hour period that "hurried" is a normal state for most.

In addition, speed in the operating room does not necessarily equate to having superior skills, despite what today's surgical culture may imply. On the surface, an unspoken belief has long existed among surgeons that speed in finishing an operation equates with being "good." Yes, having a surgeon who is fast and efficient in the operating room means less time under anesthesia for the patient. This is a good thing, *if* the speed does not create mistakes. Reckless speed in the operating room can injure or kill if the wrong surgeon is driving. Impatience can lead to carelessness, which can lead to inadvertently cutting the wrong blood vessel, perforating the intestine, or needlessly tearing organs. At times, I have been caught speeding in the operating room, and, I'm ashamed to admit, there have been patients who have paid the price. As with the inherent urge to avoid blame for mistakes, some surgeons struggle with handling the speed factor in the operating room.

How do I feel after I have not been perfect in the operating room? It is a miserable feeling knowing I inadvertently damaged a blood vessel or organ or accidentally cut a nerve. It is a sickening feeling, instantly all-consuming, paralyzing. Have I panicked in the face of a mistake? Yes. Do I know how to disguise it well in the operating room? Absolutely. If the damage is minor, the panic is short-lived. If it is major, I have to work to tighten my anal sphincter and refocus enough to repair the damage. Most patients will never know exactly what transpired in the operating room unless I decide there is a need to tell them. The only real way for any patient to understand what happened in the operating room is to read the operative note dictated by the surgeon. In deciphering the language in the legal record of your operation, you will have a better understanding of what the surgeon did.

Most patients never think of asking for a copy of their operative report. If you have questions after surgery and they go unanswered, ask your surgeon for the report. You may find the answers you seek.

In regard to Mr. Andrews's complication, my mistake in the operating room was misjudging the adequacy of his intestinal connection. His connection was not airtight and I can only speculate as to why. This type of complication, as with many created in the operating room, only surfaces later, during recovery. When Mr. Andrews returned to the emergency room, I knew right away what had happened. My initial reaction was to blame the stapling device used to make the connection. I wanted to shift the blame to something, anything other than myself. I wanted Mr. Andrews to think that I was perfect during his operation and the tools I used had been imperfect. This reaction, to shift blame when things go wrong, is instinctual and surfaces out of survival. The rigors of surgical training did not offer much sympathy for imperfection on any level. Mistakes were always a sign of weakness during training and threatened a resident's likelihood to finish the program. Today, the surgical culture is more receptive to the admission of errors and to learning from them.

In the end, I am the one solely responsible for any patient I choose to operate on. I am the one responsible for my imperfections inside and outside the operating room. Even today, I continue to struggle with admitting mistakes or misjudgments to patients and their families. I struggle because I think I should be perfect every time. I struggle because of the potential damage to my reputation and practice and the real possibility of administrative and legal punishment. Early in my career, I did not always have the maturity to accept my responsibility. With time I have come to realize that imperfection is an inherent part of my profession. I realize that the best way to explain imperfection is with honesty and sincerity. Most patients respect honesty.

Mr. Andrews did have a prolonged hospital stay as a result of his complication. He ultimately healed satisfactorily without requiring another operation and left the hospital. But he was never the same. His body and mind never truly recovered from what had occurred. It was too much of an insult on top of his initial surgery. I was never the same either. A small part of me never recovered from seeing the physical and emotional pain my patient had to endure on a daily basis for several weeks. Once he left the hospital, all I could do was file away the emotions of this experience in a small corner of my brain and wall it off. I had to; the next day I had to be ready to operate again. Mr. Andrews's face will never be forgotten. He has taken his place in the room with the others who have come before him. A room with a door that is always open.

Chapter 4

The White Coat Code of Silence

Catherine Williams was a healthy, fifty-two-year-old mother of two when she walked into a well-respected community hospital for a scheduled hysterectomy. Her gynecologist had recommended the surgery as the best way to address heavy bleeding caused by uterine fibroid tumors. As her surgeon explained, a partial hysterectomy (removal of the uterus, leaving the ovaries intact) was a routine procedure with minimal risk. (It is, as a matter of fact, one of the most commonly performed operations in America today.) Mrs. Williams was told to expect to be in the hospital for several days, after which she would continue to recover at home, returning to normal activities gradually over the next few weeks.

Things didn't go quite that way.

Before it was all said and done, Mrs. Williams would endure

a prolonged hospital stay, a damaged ureter, a colostomy, a serious infection caused by a small surgical sponge left in her abdomen after the hysterectomy, and two major operations.

I met Mrs. Williams (unintentionally) a few hours after she had entered the hospital. It was early in my career. Between operations, as I waited for setup on my second case, a distress call came from an operating room across the hall.

"We need help in here, *now*!" An O.R. door flew open. "Is there another surgeon around?" I saw the nurse for only a second before she ducked back in. I peered down the corridor. Surely other surgeons had heard the call for help, but the hall was empty. There were, apparently, no volunteers available. The lack of response seemed a little odd. Something didn't quite make sense . . . but I didn't have time to figure out what. In light of the silence, I guessed I was *it*. Immediately, I began to feel a little full of myself; there was a crisis and I was the one who would come to the rescue. It would be my first experience helping a colleague in distress, and my ego liked it. I strode briskly to the open door, peered in, and in that instant was introduced to the covert world of imperfect surgery.

Mrs. Williams was in big trouble on that operating room table. She was unconscious, paralyzed, and being kept alive by machines. Her face was swollen like a bloated tick. Blood-tinged tubes came from her nose and mouth. Her body was strapped to the operating room table and tilted toward her head to maintain blood flow to her brain. The reason: Rapid and excessive blood loss during her surgery was sending Mrs. Williams into hypovolemic shock, a condition in which the heart cannot supply the body with enough blood, initiating organ failure. The anesthesiologist at the head of her bed was frantically pumping blood into her veins as fast as she was losing it. Her abdomen was wide open. The scrub nurse didn't have enough hands to contain Mrs. Williams's intestines.

Out of the corner of my eye, I could see the recently removed uterus posing solo on an instrument table. I scrubbed quickly, gowned, gloved, and surveyed the scene. Blood was leaking from some veins deep in her pelvis, damaged during the hysterectomy. This hemorrhaging had to be stemmed right away. I could also see urine spouting from a human-made hole in her right ureter, the tube carrying urine from her kidney to her bladder. This tube runs very close to a woman's uterus and can be damaged during a hysterectomy. This hole had to be repaired quickly. Finally, I noticed fresh stool percolating from several more cuts in her left colon.

"Shit," I muttered. "I'm going to have to give this woman a colostomy." There was just too much contamination to repair her damaged colon without it, too much risk for infection. I paused and shook my head. Most patients do not take kindly to surprises after they wake up from surgery. "She is not going to like this."

I looked up at the patient's surgeon. "What a mess." I cleared my throat. "What the hell happened here?" He didn't answer. I could only surmise what had occurred during the removal of Mrs. Williams's uterus. The collateral damage was significant. I suspected that her surgeon's scalpel had strayed and significant bleeding had followed. Then, during his desperate attempt to remove the uterus as quickly as possible and stop the bleeding, he had damaged other nearby organs. My conquering-hero glow was gone. I was now pissed off at myself for volunteering, and more than a little frightened.

When unexpected, rapid bleeding occurs during a "routine" operation, it scares the shit out of any surgeon, including me. Most of us quell the panic by focusing on what needs to be done to stop the bleeding. It's a frightening time; the life is literally draining out of your patient, right before your eyes. You must make the repairs within a matter of seconds. Sometimes, grasping blindly into a rising pool of blood, in an effort to stop it with a clamp, invites more bleeding. This becomes an unnerving spiral that can end tragically. I've seen patients bleed to death on the operating room table. A hideous feeling of helplessness, mixed with denial, is followed by a profound sadness unlike any other. Every surgeon has been there at least once; some will be there again. It's the nature of our business.

When no answer came from behind the surgeon's mask, I made another quick inventory of Mrs. Williams's damaged organs. Was this scenario a recurring theme with him? If so, how could he still be performing major surgery? I knew nothing about this surgeon, nothing about his reputation. Did Mrs. Williams know anything about his operating skills? I had a lot of questions but no time for answers. This was not the time to find out who was behind the surgical mask. Now was the time to move, to get this woman off the operating room table, *alive*. With the help of my partner and another colleague, we repaired the damaged ureter and removed the injured segment of colon. Unfortunately, because of the blood loss and stool contamination, I had to give Mrs. Williams a temporary colostomy, something that could be reversed four months later.

A colostomy involves drawing the healthier end of the large

intestine (colon) through an incision in the abdomen, allowing the rest of the colon to recover from the surgery. The opening is fitted with a bag and serves as the route for the elimination of feces until the patient is sufficiently healed. Once enough time has passed, the patient can return to the operating room for a colostomy reversal, during which the bag is removed, the two ends of the colon reattached, and the incision closed.

With the damage repaired, I had to move on before Mrs. Williams's operation ended; my next scheduled patient was in the O.R. down the hall, ready for his operation. I called in one of my partners to finish the rescue. It felt good to be a surgeon that day, knowing I'd had a hand in turning around a potentially disastrous outcome.

Over the next seven days, I saw Mrs. Williams several times while she recovered in the hospital. Eventually, she was able to go home. But she wasn't home for long; two weeks later she was readmitted to the hospital with a serious intra-abdominal infection. The cause: A surgical sponge had been left in her abdomen by her surgeon.

I did not learn of Mrs. Williams's rehospitalization, however, until the day a certified letter from her attorney arrived. "Dr. Paul Ruggieri and Drs. _____ are hereby named as defendants in the lawsuit . . ." I felt like throwing up. The ink on my malpractice policy wasn't even dry and I was getting sucked into the black hole of a medical malpractice lawsuit.

As it turned out, Mrs. Williams had been readmitted to the hospital and endured yet another major operation—to remove the sponge (the cause of the infection) from her abdominal cavity. I wondered how much she knew about the *other* mistakes made during her hysterectomy, or how close she had come to dying that day. This last complication was, evidently, the straw that broke her legal back.

As the months passed and the lawsuit unfolded, I became more acquainted with Mrs. Williams's surgeon. The man looked great on paper. He had all the official qualifications to operate on humans. And he had been in practice for years. Despite his being older and wiser, though, his operating skills had been deteriorating for years and his surgical mishaps becoming more frequent. As information surfaced, I began to understand why no one else had volunteered to help him during Mrs. Williams's operation. I also began to understand why I was the first surgeon to bail him out on that fateful day. Every surgeon in the community had taken a turn answering his distress calls and cleaning up his complications, risking their reputation and livelihood. As the "new kid on the block," I had become the sacrificial lamb in the operating room that day and, ultimately, in the courtroom. I was new to the community, naïve to the reputations of the surgeons practicing at the hospital. No one had taken me aside and warned me about the surgeons I needed to be wary of. I was in the dark just as much as Mrs. Williams.

At the end of the day, I was angry at Mrs. Williams's surgeon for putting my budding reputation in jeopardy. I was just getting my feet wet as a surgeon and now had to deal with the ugliness and distraction of a malpractice lawsuit. I was also upset at my colleagues for passively hanging in the shadows while I became stained. I was angry at the hospital for allowing the man to continue to operate, despite actively "monitoring" his performance. What the hell were they monitoring? I became even more enraged during one of my depositions as the guy's lawyer attempted to spread blame.

"Dr. Ruggieri," he began. There was a long pause. "My client states that he noticed the injury to the ureter *after* you came in to help. He claims it was injured during your dissection."

I could not believe what I was hearing. "You mean to tell me that bastard is blaming me for that?" I had to get up from my chair and walk. Here I had bailed out this son of a bitch, and now he was trying to take me down with him. I sat back down. "Mr. Lawyer, the hole in the ureter was made *before* I arrived in the operating room. It was made by your client."

As the lawsuit ran its course, I became angrier. I wanted answers to why and how everyone around me had become covert enablers of a surgeon who should not have been operating. I wanted answers as to how such a "head in the sand" environment could exist in any hospital. What were the factors that allowed surgeons like this one to continue working, despite leaving behind a long and wide trail of complications and bad outcomes? Why hadn't other surgeons spoken up? Did a "white coat code of silence" exist?

In the end, despite his desperate attempts to spread blame, justice prevailed for Mrs. Williams, my partners, and me. The case against me and my partners was dismissed. Mrs. Williams's surgeon lost his privileges, and, fortunately for future patients, he would never see the inside of an operating room again. But there was still a cost to be paid: For the next ten years I would have to explain on every hospital or state license application why

I was brought into the lawsuit. Today, I am still angry and searching for answers. I can only wonder if Mrs. Williams found any after her ordeal.

/ / /

The "white coat code of silence" is a term I use to describe the dark side of a profession that, despite its noble intentions, enables incompetent surgeons to continue to work. It's a culture that originates during the training years of residency and is currently characterized by complacency, fear, and a lack of confidence. There is a complacency, a reluctance among surgeons to speak up and draw attention to themselves. There is fear of a legal system that may "entrap" them. There is also a lack of confidence in the current systems hospitals have set up to deal with incompetence. Most surgeons do not want to complicate their professional, legal, and personal lives by painting themselves as whistleblowers. For that matter, who does?

This code of silence is not obvious in the surgical world, not something you can reference or directly measure. It is a subtle, subconscious pressure that many fine physicians succumb to despite the best intentions. This code of silence has proven to be resilient, largely because of apathy. In the past, my profession has not done a good job of policing its own. Why are surgeons who are known to be dangerous allowed to continue to operate independently, under the radar, despite colleagues' concerns about skills and complication rates? Where is the oversight? Why couldn't Mrs. Williams have known more about her surgeon's record? How in the world could she be expected to make an informed decision about his competency without access to information about his history of performance?

///

The origins of this professional silence are rooted in the experiences and indoctrinations of a surgeon's training years—or at least that was true for me and most of my peers. I trained in an era, and at an institution, where the old-guard attitude was the prevailing dogma. By "old guard," I mean working until you drop, shouldering blame, and speaking only when spoken to. Today, most surgical training programs are kinder and gentler on many fronts (including the hours). When I was a surgical resident, the opportunity to learn the secrets of surgery from my mentors came at a hefty price, paid in blood (literally, at times), humiliation, tears, and chronic sleep deprivation. During my time as a lowly intern/resident, my work ethic was motivated mostly by fear of failure. I was petrified of screwing up because I knew the blame would come down like a hammer. As an underling, if something went wrong or a patient did not do well, I was to blame. No questions asked. Failure morphed into fear, the fear of looking bad or losing a job. Today, there is even more at risk for me, because failure can turn into a death or a lawsuit.

Of course, all blame flowed from the top down. The acrimony would flow from the attending surgeon, who would blame the chief resident, who would in turn blame the intern. It was a musical chairs of blame with the lowest person left without a chair when the music stopped. The intense conditions coupled with the teaching were a rite of passage. You had to take it or get out. I took it; not all my colleagues did. Amazingly, many of my mentors trained under even more hellish circumstances, which only reinforced their teaching methods. Their motto was, "This is how I did it, so this is how you will do it."

One of my most infamous mentors cursed constantly and blamed me for *everything*. The best I could do was grin and take it. Period. There was no questioning his authority if I wanted to become a surgeon. I had no voice, no leverage. I had nothing. Hell, he could have blamed me for the Kennedy assassination and I would have admitted being in Dealey Plaza in Dallas on November 22, 1963. What choice did I have? None whatsoever. I conformed to what my mentors demanded. I desperately wanted to be a surgeon and did whatever had to be done.

During those years, I learned to shut up and not draw attention to myself. Garnering attention, in any fashion, was not met with positive reinforcement. I went about my business with blinders on, purposely unaware of any imperfection around me. I had neither the time nor interest to pay attention to the successes or shortcomings of the guy next to me. He or she was not my problem, and I had my own to attend to. I also learned that blame was part of the culture and even today, I have to work at not dispensing it needlessly. The attitudes I was exposed to during training have left an imprint that I've carried to every operating room I have ever worked in. For me, it has been difficult to wash away the stains of training because they were such an integral part of my professional fabric.

In training, we learn to strive constantly for perfection. Failure to achieve it is not acceptable and certainly not talked about. Adhering to this mind-set contributes to the development of the white coat code of silence in the next generation of surgeons. When I was a surgeon in training, my ego said failure was *never* an option because of the real-life human consequences associated with it. When mistakes were made, patients got hurt or died. I *had* to be perfect. Intense working conditions, adversity, and imperfect human coworkers—these were not acceptable excuses. And, as time went by, I acquiesced and viewed failures as someone else's problem. (Obviously, this was not always true.) The problem, I found, was balancing my growing ego with the consequences of failures. Some of us hid our weaknesses with the same intense determination we showed toward our work. If I could not face my own imperfections, how in the world could I even approach a discussion of another surgeon's failures? As a surgeon about to enter practice, I carried these attitudes with me. They were an inescapable part of my past and it would be difficult to pull away from them.

/ / /

He that is without sin, cast the first stone.
—JOHN 8

I had to do something drastic to stop Dr. V from continuing to operate. I could not keep my head in the sand any longer. The evidence was mounting and too many people were not getting proper surgical care.

I suspected that most of my surgical colleagues were becoming aware (even if only generally) of Dr. V's less than stellar operative history. Hospitals are small worlds unto themselves, and it does not take long for the staff to know everyone's work. The operating rooms are even more insular; there, secrets are often not openly discussed, rarely going beyond the double doors. Operating room nurses quickly figure out which surgeons know what they're doing and which ones should be looking for another profession.

Most of the operating room nurses were familiar with Dr. V's body of work but dared not openly complain. To hospitals, surgeons are sacrosanct because of the revenue they generate. To most operating room nurses, surgeons are considered king of the hill, untouchable. This attitude is especially pervasive among older nurses, many of whom still place surgeons on a pedestal despite long records of imperfections. In the case of Dr. V, the best the nurses could do was pass along anonymous handwritten notes (one did have the courage to sign his name) detailing their concerns to the chief of surgery—me.

In some ways, surgeons are like professional athletes. They have been held in such high esteem their entire careers that not many people are comfortable questioning their authority or skills. As time passed, not *one* surgeon in the community expressed any concerns regarding the continued complications of Dr. V. I do not fault them for this. There was a lot at stake for them professionally to speak out openly against a colleague. Surgeons are not supposed to criticize other surgeons. It isn't part of the code. It was as if he did not exist. Yet at the end of every month, I was reminded that he *did* exist, when the monthly report on complications of all the hospital's surgeons would come across my desk.

As chief of surgery, I was in a position of authority and it was up to me to decide how to proceed. Frankly, I was not sure how to deal with the situation since I had never been down this road before. As I gathered data to support what would be my ultimate decision, I examined the potential negative consequences of taking a stand. One of my biggest fears was the threat of legal action. I had seen this before in other communities. I could envision a lawsuit brought against me, or the hospital I represented, for what lawyers called "restraint of trade." It did not help the fact that I, and the group I belonged to, were his direct competition in the community. I could hear the lawyers now. Talk about a potential conflict of interest. I could see how this could be used against me, especially by his supporters (and he did have them). His supporters were other physicians within his large multi-specialty group who were linked to him financially. They were physicians who believed whatever he wanted them to believe.

It was bad enough that I had to worry about the potential threat of lawsuits from my patients; now I had to worry about being sued by another surgeon. Doctors suing doctors is never pretty, especially when it makes the newspapers. The quagmire of legal action is a real threat in preventing other surgeons in any community from making any type of legitimate statement against someone whose work is clearly hurting patients. It usually appears to be all about ego and money. I was not happy with how this was unfolding.

Another real concern I had about speaking up was the fear of losing business and referrals. The reality of private practice is that, to make a living, I rely on referrals from primary care physicians. I am a surgeon, a specialist. My patients come from other doctors who know my work and trust me to take care of their patients. Ideally, this referral pattern is based on experience and trust. It takes a while to build this trust, and as a young associate, I just wanted to keep my mouth shut and work. Dr. V belonged to a multispecialty group in town. It was a group whose primary care doctors continued to refer patients to me because my work spoke for itself. If I were to take a negative stand against one of their own, my referrals from the physicians in Dr. V's group would dry up. I could see his group circling its wagons and hitting me where it hurt—in the wallet. They had their weapons and would not be afraid to use them. The cold financial realities of private practice were complicating my decision.

As the months passed and more of Dr. V's patients experienced complications, I knew something had to give. I knew I was getting close to making a decision by the dwindling hours of sleep I got each night. Every morning my heart told me I had to take a stand. I was chief of surgery and I had to say something. Then, my brain would shout, *It's not worth it to stick your neck out. He is not your problem. He is the hospital's problem. Let them deal with it!*

It would have been very easy for me to allow this issue to pass. I could have paid it lip service and bided my time. Throughout the process, I consulted with hospital administrators who were in positions to support me about what I believed should be done. They were in complete agreement but let me know I would have to be the first to get the process going. As chief of the department, I was the legitimate voice. But even with their backing, I was still reluctant to speak up.

Several more weeks had gone by when it was brought to my attention that Dr. V's privileges were coming up for renewal. As chief of surgery, I had to sign those privileges, a signature that would allow him to practice for another two years. I soon would be at the crossroads of a decision. During the interim, I tried to block out this problem, hoping it would go away. It was easy to block out anything unpleasant, given the workload of my job. At night, though, when things calmed down, it would always resurface. *Why me? Why do I have to stick my neck out? Everyone knows this guy needs to go. Why do I have to be the one to take the hit?*

As I lay awake at night, worrying, I thought about how the healthcare community would feel when they found out about the decision. I thought about being labeled a whistleblower or a troublemaker. I wondered how other doctors I worked with would feel once they learned I had made a decision that negatively impacted a colleague, a surgeon. Would I be an outcast? Surgeons (much like police officers, lawyers, and other professionals) are not supposed to go against their own. Our struggles through the training years have supposedly solidified our comradeship for life. It is not in our nature to turn on ourselves. Studies have looked at this phenomenon (including one from Harvard Medical School), focusing on physicians troubled by alcohol, drug abuse, or incompetency. The Harvard study surveyed American physicians and found that 17 percent had direct knowledge of an incompetent or impaired physician. It also found that 33 percent of those with direct knowledge had not reported it to anyone in authority. The conclusions revealed that doctors are reluctant to report a colleague to the appropriate hospital authorities because "nothing will get done" and they would have stuck their neck out for no reason. Other frequently cited reasons included "It is someone else's problem" and "I don't want to risk the possibility of retribution." Today, the environment is not ripe enough to persuade doctors, especially surgeons, to speak up.

At this point, I was not ready to speak up.

Several more weeks passed and the deadline approached. I was resolute about what my heart wanted to do but hesitated because of what my brain was telling me. To sit in judgment of someone else's imperfections was daunting and very much an exercise in introspection. I was looking in a mirror, looking at myself, facing my own imperfections. Any surgeon will admit (well, at least the ones I know) that he or she is not perfect. We all have had our complications, our mistakes in and out of the operating room. We all have caused undue pain and suffering along the road of treating patients. When I looked at Dr. V's imperfections, I had to reflect on my own. "He that is without sin, cast the first stone," echoed in my head. I, too, had "sinned." How could I cast a stone?

As the weeks went by and I ruminated on my choices, one point continued to rest in the pit of my stomach. The number and seriousness of Dr. V's imperfections were far above anyone else's in the community, and this was not going to change. In the end, my decision was based on the need to protect the safety of patients. As chief of surgery, I was obligated to make that my first concern.

The day arrived. I had already been to the bathroom three times before the big eight A.M. meeting, which would be attended by all the department chiefs and clinical administrators. I had no idea what the reaction was going to be, and, at this point, I did not care. I took my seat quietly, sitting next to two individuals whom I could count on for support. When the moment arrived for me to comment on Dr. V's privileges, I stood up. My undershirt was sticking to me and my legs were shaking. "I have reviewed the available data and have concluded I cannot sign my name approving this man's operating privileges."

A collective gasp, which soon morphed into loud protests from his supporters, immediately filled the room. My legs weakened, but I continued on, giving my reasons. It was the longest ten minutes of my life.

Some in the room were shocked by my proclamation, especially those with financial links to Dr. V's practice. Others welcomed it. I knew that by using this forum, I would be able to get people's attention. I was the chief of surgery, and my words that day opened eyes.

The months that followed were filled with meetings with administrators, meetings with lawyers, and more meetings with lawyers. Dr. V had lawyers because my proclamation threatened his reputation and livelihood. The hospital had lawyers to push the recommendation forward. Lawyers were everywhere. The funny thing was, I never had to get a lawyer. Once I pulled the scab off this festering sore, the *hospital* had to do something. During the legal wrangling, I left the scene; after my term as chief expired, I chose to slide back into practicing surgery only. I was fed up with the lawyers, the egos, and just wanted to be left alone to deal with the repercussions of my decision.

My words did not immediately result in any changes. They did, however, shine some light on the dark side of my profession. After my unorthodox declaration, Dr. V's practice limped along for a few more years. He ultimately succumbed to market forces (and forces within his own group) and left the area in search of a job in another community. I wondered how someone like this could begin work in another community, leaving his past behind. In the end, after all the lawyers' meetings, all the threats, and all the worrying, the community was a safer place. And, eventually, I returned to sleeping soundly at night.

For several years, I spoke to no one about my thoughts during the ordeal. When I did revisit the experience, it was in the context of a conversation with a colleague about transparency in the surgical profession. We were performing a colon resection together. "Why did you stick your neck out like that? He wasn't your problem. With competition like that, who needs advertising?" My colleague smiled.

"He *was* my problem. He was *everyone's* problem. The sad thing was that his patients had no idea who they were getting as a surgeon. How does anyone who is about to have surgery truly know how competent the surgeon is? How can the public know? It *is* up to us to be vigilant in policing our own. If we don't do it effectively, someone else will. If it were up to me, I would make everything public knowledge. I would make public all our performance records, good and bad. Let the public decide whom to choose as a surgeon."

"You did the right thing." A pause. "Nurse, clamp please." With one quick hand motion, the diseased segment of colon was gone for good.

The culture I trained in, and continue to practice in, is complex. When it comes to being honest about another colleague or myself, there are gray areas of decision making that I truly want to avoid. Despite this, attitudes and practice climates are improving. They are improving because of a change in the culture of blame that many health professionals (especially surgeons) believe is a risk to their livelihood. This change all started with the publication of a landmark paper that sent shock waves through the medical profession.

In 1999, the Institute of Medicine published *To Err Is Human: Building a Safer Health System*. Since its publication, the health-care system in this country has never been the same. This study, a first of its kind, looked at data from hospitals across the country and concluded that 44,000 to 98,000 deaths occurred in hospitals each year from medical errors—an astounding finding. Despite statistical questions on how the data was collected and interpreted, the report exposed the public to what many in my profession suspected. Regardless of its flaws, the study was the first of its kind, and its impact was felt immediately. The raw numbers were shocking. They became a battle cry for more transparency and change in the healthcare system.

It came as no shock to me that someone had finally put a number on the imperfections of everyone (nurses and doctors) working in the healthcare system. Yes, doctors (especially surgeons, because of what they do) are human, and capable of making mistakes. When mistakes are made, people get hurt or die. In the past (and present), when patients got hurt or died from mistakes, patients' families were left with a lot of unanswered questions. In the past (and still today), the saying "Doctors bury their mistakes" had some credence to it. Even recent autopsy studies have concluded that between 8 and 24 percent of hospital deaths resulting from a major error in diagnosis get buried.

To Err Is Human began a process of peeling away the outer layer of the white coat code of silence. It exposed the good and bad of my workplace. It set the tone for an honest dialogue in a profession that had been mute for a very long time. Surgeons, myself included, were initially taken aback by the sheer weight of the numbers of patients affected. The study forced us to look in the mirror and reexamine ourselves, our attitudes, and our mechanisms for monitoring safety. It forced all involved in the delivery of healthcare to refocus on improving efforts to deliver safe, quality care. The doors for transparency were busted wide open by *To Err Is Human*. The winds of change were about to sweep through my profession. I would either embrace and ride these winds or get blown away by them.

As the years followed, I saw the acceptance of change and transparency in surgery firsthand. Before the publication of this study, for example, it was unusual to see an article in the surgical literature examining the etiology of surgeons' mistakes inside the operating room. Studies on this topic were rarely undertaken, and never openly discussed or published for the public and press to consume. When they were discussed, it was behind closed doors. Today, scientific articles published by the Harvards and Mayo Clinics of the medical world analyzing surgical mistakes are showing up in reputable surgical journals with frequency. Many are written in an effort to educate and add to the transparency spurred on by *To Err Is Human*.

Prior to the publication of *To Err Is Human*, all hospitals in this country had a system in place to evaluate the outcomes (both good and bad) of individual surgeons on a routine basis. This process, known as peer review, consists of monthly meetings during which recent surgical complications and deaths are discussed with the hope of learning what happened and how to prevent it from occurring again. These meetings have traditionally been a forum for surgeons to openly discuss why things went wrong with our patients. For the most part, the conversations are cordial and educational. Early in my career, I often found it intimidating to openly explain to my colleagues why a specific patient of mine had suffered a complication or even died. It was not easy to openly admit your mistakes or misjudgments to others. As my career advanced, I become more comfortable with my admissions at these meetings. Yet even now, I still have to swallow hard before admitting to "an error in judgment" or "a technical error in the operating room."

The discussions and conclusions reached in the peer review process are legally protected from being used as evidence in malpractice courts of law. This is comforting but does not lessen the blow to the ego when you take center stage. The information revealed at these meetings is used internally to monitor bad outcomes of all surgeons. It is a required forum in all hospitals and a necessary step in the arduous process of addressing a surgeon who does not measure up to the standard of care.

The release of *To Err Is Human* dramatically influenced the peer review process and how it evaluated all physicians, especially surgeons. The study tried to set an honest tone for transparency so physicians would not feel threatened about admitting and learning from their mistakes. In the aftermath of *To Err Is Human*, the stakes surrounding the peer review process were raised dramatically, because hospitals came under pressure to come up with better standardized methods to minimize the risk of errors and complications associated with patient care. Much of this pressure revolved around getting paid: In the aftermath of this study, the federal government and insurance companies chose not to reimburse hospitals for the costs of certain mistakes and complications that undermined the quality of care of hospitalized patients. These included healthcare costs incurred by patients who accidentally fell while in the hospital, intravenous catheter infections acquired in the hospital, pressure ulcers acquired in the hospital, and costs associated with wrong-site surgery, to name a few. The new mantra was, *Find ways to improve the quality of care; prevent complications and mistakes or you will not get paid.* Health insurance companies (and the federal government) were empowered to use the statistic of 44,000 to 98,000 unnecessary deaths each year as the impetus to improve the quality of care, reduce errors, and reduce costs.

As a direct result of the information and changes brought forward by *To Err Is Human*, the peer review process has taken on a more serious tone. Today, there are more criteria for reporting serious complications, errors, and deaths to state review medical boards than in the past. Unexpected patient deaths are discussed and automatically scrutinized by more hospital committees than ever before. More patient cases are being sent outside the hospital walls for an independent review of the quality of care given.

What the public does *not* know is that hospitals today are

keenly aware of the track record of every surgeon operating within their walls. Our complication rates and infection rates are constantly monitored. In addition, hospitals provide quarterly updates on key quality measures: surgical patients' length of stay in the hospital, how often patients are brought back to the operating room to address a complication of the original surgery, and how often patients are readmitted to the hospital after they are initially discharged. In years past, much of the outcome data was never discussed openly with the respective surgeons. I intuitively knew, just as your surgeon knows, what my complication rate was for removing someone's gallbladder. Now, I see it in black and white on a report every quarter. A report for my eyes only.

Today, every surgeon at every hospital is continually made aware of how he or she is performing with respect to his or her peers. In addition, the insurance companies that write out the checks are also aware of how individual surgeons are performing.

This new "transparency" is all good, but the public is still completely unaware of what the hospital's files reveal on surgeons in its community. There is no Web site, no ability to research important, relevant data on your surgeon's track record before your operation. All you know are two things: Your primary care physician referred you to this particular surgeon, and he or she has a "good" reputation. Is this enough? Hospitals have relevant information. Insurance companies have it as well. Even your surgeon has it in his or her head. The mother of three about to have her gallbladder removed has no way of knowing how her surgeon's complication rates compare to those of the surgeon across town. Today, she has no way of acquiring hard data on her surgeon's track record. The one exception to this involves cardiac surgeons. A number of states now publish public data on individual heart surgeons' performance, revealing complication rates and death rates. Today, all the mother of three can rely on is her own doctor's trust in the surgeon ready to remove her gallbladder.

I believe every person who is about to undergo surgery should have the opportunity to access unbiased performance information about his or her surgeon. What's important? The number of operations that surgeon has performed, his or her complication rates, his or her patients' length of stay in the hospital, mortality rates, and patient satisfaction surveys. I believe that eventually there will be periodic public report cards for every surgeon in this country, outlining meaningful data that prospective patients can use to make a choice. The days of surgeons and hospitals keeping quiet on performance data are over.

Most of the surgeons I know are skilled, caring individuals who are proud of their work. They would not shy away from having clear, easy-to-understand performance data available for the public. In the future, in the name of improving quality, surgeons will have no choice but to allow the public access to vital data; they will not get paid otherwise. We are in a new era of transparency in medicine, mainly driven by the influential organizations that want to improve quality and reduce costs. These groups believe the time has come for the public to have access to legitimate data before stepping into the operating room—the good and bad of what we do—and I agree. The edges of the white coat code of silence are fraying.

Chapter 5

Get Out of My Operating Room

"This thing is a piece of shit. Get it the hell out of my operating room!" The colon stapling device exploded into pieces when I hurled it against the operating room wall. I was fed up with its failure to work as advertised by the manufacturer. The stapler had probably cost less than $100 to make. The hospital paid $300 for it (and then billed the patient, or insurance company, $1,200). Now the thing didn't even work.

I do not react well to imperfection inside the operating room. I cannot tolerate it in the tools I use, the staff assisting me, or myself. Defective devices—I can have them replaced. Unmotivated staff—I can have them removed from the operating room. I haven't quite figured out what to do with myself yet.

Surgeons are control freaks. We have to be. And when things don't go our way in the operating room, we can have outbursts. Some of us curse, some throw instruments, others have tantrums. These explosions are a go-to reaction when we're confronted with the ghosts of prior complications. The nonfunctioning stapler had transported me to a specter of an operation past.

Several months earlier, I had performed the same operation on a sixty-six-year-old patient, using an identical stapling device. Everything seemed to have worked perfectly until the patient developed severe complications four days after his surgery. We soon discovered the cause: the nonperformance of the stapling device.

When the stapler hit the wall, I had been in the operating room for more than four hours, struggling to remove a diseased segment of colon from Mr. Baker, a 330-pound middle-aged man. Trying to keep his fat out of my way during the operation had been a continuous battle. The pain in my upper back reminded me that I was losing the fight.

Obese patients create more physical work for a surgeon during *any* type of procedure. Operations take longer in obese patients, lead to surgeon fatigue and frustration, and leave our upper body in knots. And obese patients automatically face an increased risk of complications such as infection, pneumonia, and blood clots during recovery as well. Surgeons know this. So why do we take them on as patients? With more than a third of the American population now obese, we literally can't be that selective.

In addition to the difficulty Mr. Baker's obesity was causing, there had been a steady loss of blood during the case. I was not happy with how things were going. It seemed whatever I touched bled. His tissue reacted to the slightest graze with more bleeding. I didn't know how to break the cycle.

Why does this guy have to bleed like this? As if it were his fault. Here I was blaming him. Hell, *I* was the one causing the bleeding. But in surgery, it always has to be someone else's fault. It's never the surgeon's fault.

"Can someone help me here, please? I can't see a damn thing."

Surgeons hate for a patient to lose blood during an operation. They hate it because dealing with bleeding adds more work to the case, adds time to the operation, interferes with perfection, and can lead to mistakes. Ureters, nerves, organs, and more blood vessels than you can imagine get cut accidentally when excessive bleeding can't be controlled. The surgeon literally cannot see well enough when the field keeps filling with blood. The other reason surgeons hate excessive blood loss is that it's a reflection of their operative skills. In the dark corners of operating rooms, we whisper about surgeons who lose excessive amounts of blood during routine operations. It is never talked about openly, but the gossip is heard in our tightly sealed world.

Interestingly, most surgeons tend to underestimate the blood loss after an operation. They can't help themselves. "I *couldn't* have lost that much blood. Impossible." Whether it's ego or denial, the reality is that blood loss can be measured, accurately, and surgeons can't hide from the numbers. Hospitals know who is losing blood, and how much, during every operation. They have data on every surgeon using their operating rooms, but the public cannot access this information. This information matters, too; in the end, a large amount of blood lost during an operation can be a harbinger of complications to come.

Surgeons, like poker players, are sometimes only as good in the operating room as the patients they are dealt. Obesity, excessive scar tissue from a previous surgery in the same area, disease that is more advanced than anticipated—any of these physiological conditions create more work and a more difficult environment for the surgeon. And underlying or chronic conditions such as a history of hypertension, cardiac disease, or lung disease immediately put patients at risk for complications before the surgery even begins. Today, based on your medical history, surgeons can usually analyze, quite accurately, your risk of complications (or death) before stepping foot in the operating room. All you have to do is ask.

I had no idea how bad Mr. Baker's colon disease would be until I opened him up and looked inside. It was a mess. If I were playing poker and this man's anatomy were the hand dealt, it would be time to fold.

"Son of a bitch. That is one of the ugliest pieces of colon I've ever seen." I grabbed the scrub nurse's hand. "See, touch that thing. Look how inflamed it is." Scrub nurses love to touch organs in the operating room when given the chance. "Okay, don't poke it too hard, it will start to bleed again." Her hand recoiled back onto the instrument stand. I was in for a long night.

Tonight, the diseased colon on the menu was angry, cursing and taunting me. "Good luck, Mr. Big-Time Surgeon, trying to remove me." Was I the only one in the room hearing this? Surgeons frequently have conversations with body parts or organs they are trying to remove. They also have conversations with themselves; it's a way to blow off steam while your mind scrambles to deal with the unexpected.

"By the time you are done with me, your back muscles are going to be in a heap of pain." I continued to listen. "I know what you are thinking. If my man here weren't so fat, you would have had me out of here an hour ago." The colon went on, "Looking forward to that drive home in your new Porsche? Well, tough shit. It's going to have to wait. You better take your time or I'll come back to haunt you in a few days." I could hear the colon laughing at me. I was crying inside.

"Nurse, hand me a curved scissors." Finally, I was granted a little success in freeing up one end of the colon. But that was short-lived. More bleeding. *Shit. I hate this.* And I had cut myself. I stared at my finger. "Nurse, I need a new glove." The outer skin under my glove was breached, but not deeply.

"Almost got you." I could not shut the thing up. "How do you know I don't have hepatitis or H.I.V.?"

Just great, I thought. *Now I have something else to worry about.*

"You are going to earn your fee tonight, Dr. Surgeon." The colon kept talking. "I hope you are not in this business for the money, like the last guy who operated on me. Between what Medicare pays you for this operation, the phone calls in the middle of night, and the time you spend guiding my recovery, I figure you will make about two hundred dollars an hour for this operation. How does that grab you?" It would not stop talking. I was losing patience.

Should have gone for my M.B.A., I mumbled to myself. *Big mistake going into medicine, never mind surgery. If I could only go back and do it over again.*

"Wait, subtract what it costs you in overhead personnel to bill for this operation (double that if the claim gets rejected), plus malpractice costs for the day, and we are now at a hundred fifty an hour." The rant continued. "How could I leave out the biggest expense of all? How could I forget the price it costs you (and your family) in mental stress from worrying about me after the surgery (double this cost if a complication arises)? Now, I figure you are under a hundred dollars an hour. Plumbers make more than that just to step inside your house. I bet they sleep well at night. Just remember, Dr. Surgeon, nobody put a gun to your head. You chose this profession." I could swear the thing was laughing at me. "Forget about keeping those dinner reservations tonight. You and me, we're going for breakfast once this is over."

Was this diseased segment of colon really talking to me? Anything is possible inside the operating room. The nurses may think we're crazy, but most of us have these conversations to keep our sanity. As a general surgeon, I often have a conversation with an acutely inflamed appendix as I laparoscopically remove it. Most of these are friendly chats because most appendix operations are low maintenance, low stress, fast, and lucrative.

On the other hand, a conversation with an acutely inflamed gallbladder can turn ugly as soon as the operation does. Get into some brisk bleeding in the liver bed while taking the gallbladder out and see how fast personalities change. I admit to barking at diseased segments of colon, or sweet-talking a cancerous thyroid gland away from the delicate nerves behind it (nerves that, if damaged, will cause a patient's voice to become permanently hoarse). If I'm worried about the way the dissection is going, I may even bring my malpractice lawyer into the O.R. "chat room."

Cardiac surgeons often speak to the hearts they are operating on, encouraging their muscle contractions when getting off the bypass pump machine. "Pump time" is the amount of time a patient is on the heart-lung machine during open-heart bypass surgery. It is during this time that cardiac surgeons are working quickly to suture and bypass diseased coronary arteries while the heart is not beating. Prolonged pump times (approaching three hours), during which the heart remains lifeless, can lead to an increased frequency of life-threatening complications after heart bypass surgery. Like intraoperative bleeding, a cardiac surgeon's pump time can be quietly considered an indirect measure of his or her surgical abilities. A shorter pump time equates to a better outcome. Whisperings in any cardiac surgery operating room link shorter pump times (presumably) to faster and better surgeons.

Urologic surgeons love to talk dirty to a cancerous prostate gland as they are robotically extricating it from its secluded location, deep in a man's pelvis. They need to watch out for delicate nerves, the ones that control a man's ability to have an erection and control urine flow. Impotency and urine incontinence are the major complications of prostate surgery. Urologic surgeons often quietly measure their own operating skills by their patients' post-op erectile dysfunction (E.D.) and incontinence rates.

Orthopedic surgeons, encased in their "moon walk" attire,

berate the diseased joints they are removing as the bone chips fly. Once in, the berating turns to chanting in an attempt to ward off the evil spirits of infection. Joint infection is an orthopedic surgeon's worst nightmare. Like blood loss, cardiac bypass pump times, and impotency and incontinence rates, joint infection rates are a measure of surgical performance. All of these benchmarks exist in hospital records and in each surgeon's mind. Yet patients often have no practical access to them.

Surgeons will curse at organs for being difficult or flatter them for being cooperative. One minute a diseased organ can be as seductive as a mistress; the next it can annoy the hell out of you, like a mother-in-law who has overstayed her welcome.

"I am not getting any younger. Let's get this over with." The colon's conversation with me finally ended and the room went silent. I stuck my right hand out. "Nurse, knife, please."

As the operation progressed, I came close to accidentally cutting Mr. Baker's ureter. The colon felt like a piece of wood, cemented in place. Ever try to free a piece of cemented wood from its location? Something usually tears; pieces break off or go flying. So much for perfection.

Throughout the operation, my pager had been going off without a break; I had three consults to see and one patient sitting in the emergency room with a hot appendix. The dinner reservations I had made earlier in the week with my wife for that night were as useless as the instrument I'd flung against the wall. I was beat, had to pee, and was ready for a glass of single malt. My patient was on the table with his abdomen filleted open and I wanted to be somewhere else.

"See how cheap they make these things," I said, glaring at the biggest piece of the shattered stapling device lying at my feet.

Not a soul in the room had uttered a word at my outrage, but I could sense the unease among the operating room nurses. They had never seen this type of behavior from me before. Even today, despite all the outside intrusions, a surgeon is still king in the operating room. When the king becomes vocal, everyone stops, listens, and ducks. It can get very uncomfortable when a surgeon's violent impulses erupt.

The silence in the room was quickly broken by the ringing of the phone on the wall. The nurse picked it up, listened for a moment, and turned to me. "Dr. Ruggieri, they need you in the emergency room now. A car just dropped off some guy with an open entrance wound to the abdomen. He's bleeding and some of his intestines are poking out through the hole." The nurse looked at me, waiting for an answer.

I had to pause. "Nurse," I said, biting my lip. Suddenly, a piece of fat the size of a golf ball hit the floor. It became airborne when, to emphasize my answer, I had extracted my right hand from deep inside Mr. Baker's abdomen. The yellow glob landed next to a jagged piece of colon stapler on the floor. "I am tied up here for at least another hour. Tell the emergency room doctor to call another surgeon or send the patient down the road to the city hospital."

"But, Dr. Ruggieri," the nurse holding the phone pleaded, "the man is bleeding from a hole in his abdomen. What do you want the E.R. doctor to do?"

"Put his finger in it and hold pressure." I kicked the piece of fat under the table. My dog, Chase, would have loved to chew on that.

I had finally finished removing the diseased segment of colon and was trying to connect the two ends deep in Mr. Baker's open pelvis. It was a difficult dissection because of his excess size and small pelvis (women have wide, user-friendly pelvises when it comes to colorectal surgery). Most surgeons use a colonic stapling device to reconnect the bowel. Within seconds, I can get it into position, line up the two ends of colon, pull the trigger, and be done with it. When it works, it is fast, efficient, and effective. The stapling device should create an airtight colonic connection for patients, allowing for normal bowel movements upon recovery. When the device misfires, it is a surgeon's—and patient's—worst nightmare. A defective staple line seal can leak (after the patient has been closed up and sent to a room) and lead to a serious infection, a second operation, and much angst. It can even lead to death.

My patient, Mr. Baker, was a fifty-five-year-old accountant with recurrent diverticulitis. Diverticulosis is an extremely common disease of the colon in the United States, a direct result of the American diet of low-fiber, high-fat foods coupled with a sedentary lifestyle. The disease involves the presence of small pouches in the colon wall, pouches that are potential weak spots for infection and rupture. With some patients, these pouches fill with stool, become infected, and cause intense pain. When a patient has an infection in these pouches, the disease is called diverticulitis. It's not only painful; it can make a person very ill. Diverticulitis usually responds to intravenous antibiotics and several days in the hospital. When a patient has continued bouts of infection, surgery becomes an option to prevent further relapses.

Before his surgery, during a consultation in my office, Mr. Baker made sure to tell me how much he enjoyed spending "quality time" on the toilet reading the financial section of the newspaper. The man would trade stocks on his laptop while in *the bathroom*. He shared this with me, boasting about his "toilet gains," after I informed him of the small risk that his surgery could result in a colostomy. I thought of this conversation now, in the operating room. I could not deprive Mr. Baker of his "toilet trades" by fouling up his operation, leaving him with a colostomy.

As luck would have it, the stapling device misfired badly, creating a defective seal. I had one more chance to make this right before running out of rectum. Mr. Baker was edging closer to a permanent colostomy bag; if the device misfired a second time, that would be the only option. The last thing you want your patient to find, unexpectedly, is a colostomy bag attached to his skin when he comes out of anesthesia. What would I tell Mr. Baker? His trading days on the toilet would be over. "I am so sorry but you have a permanent colostomy bag because this cheap stapling device misfired." How would I be able to face him?

Fortunately, I was able to avoid this catastrophe with a new stapling device (same kind) that did work. Maybe I hadn't lined the ends up right? Maybe there was too much tissue in between the ends of the device? Maybe the thing was defective? Why this one worked, only the surgical gods know.

/ / /

"Mrs. Baker, your husband is fine," I said into the phone. I slumped down onto a stool behind me, almost falling off the edge. "Everything went well. He will be in the recovery room for an hour before going up to his room." I could feel my bladder exploding.

"Dr. Ruggieri, I was getting worried. Why did it take so long?" she asked.

"Well." I paused for a few seconds, staring down at the blood on my shoe covers. I had to think about my answer. The wrong words can come back to haunt you. "Your husband is a large man and his disease was worse than anticipated. It just took a little longer to complete the operation." I took a deep breath. "He is doing fine." I glared at the bloodied segment of colon nestled in the plastic specimen bucket.

"Thank you, Dr. Ruggieri." Mrs. Baker was relieved.

I hung up the phone, thinking about what I had just said. Should I have told her more? Now, the worrying begins and it will not end until Mr. Baker leaves the hospital. It begins because I know in my heart this operation did *not* go smoothly. Not every operation does. Not every surgeon has his or her A game on for every case, for whatever reason. Not every patient is the ideal patient, ideal enough to make my job easier, to make perfection easier. I can perform the same operation on two different patients on the same day and have two opposite experiences. How does this happen? It happens because every human being's anatomy is unique and every person's disease is different. It happens because a perfect first operation does not guarantee a perfect second operation. It happens because my hand may deviate and accidentally cut into something else. It happens because I cannot re-create the exact same movements every time, during every operation, with every patient. It happens because I may be in a hurry and get careless. It happens because human beings make mistakes when stressed, fatigued, or distracted. It happens because the moon may be full and Lady Luck may only have time to stick around for the operation preceding yours. Every operation I perform comes with an asterisk in front of it. Remember, past performances do not guarantee future returns.

After one of these "perfect" operations, I feel like standing in the operating room doorway, arms outstretched, shouting, "I am king of the world!" It feels that good. As a surgeon, I expect to experience perfection every time I step into the operating room. There are no worries attached to perfection. No insomnia, no gray hairs. No checking the limits on my malpractice policy.

A surgeon knows the potential consequences of every event, both good and bad, that occurs during an operation. In the end, surgeons carefully judge what to tell (or not tell) family members about the details of a case. A surgeon has to decide what to worry a patient's family with and what to leave out. Families do not need to know every detail of an operation unless the surgeon judges it important for the patient's recovery. At the end of an operation, the surgeon dictates a report that includes all the details of what transpired. It is part of the legal medical record and can be made available to anyone who has surgery. If a patient has questions, the answers should be in the operative report. This report describes the findings, any problems encountered, and how they were corrected. It does *not* tell the story of how hard your surgeon worked, how he or she felt after the surgery, or if there were any near misses.

Mrs. Baker will never know what my heart felt like after her husband's surgery. From a technical point of view, this was not an A-plus operation on my part. I would give it an A for effort but B-minus for quality. Overall, it gets an E because I was exhausted. I did the best I could under the circumstances. I left the operating room with a sour feeling in my gut, in addition to the pain in my neck. I left worrying that Mr. Baker's obesity, his badly diseased colon, the prolonged operation, the mess with the misfired stapler, and extensive blood loss put him at risk for complications during his hospital recovery.

When Mr. Baker leaves the hospital, all he will see is a fresh scar on his abdomen. When he is in the bathroom selling stocks, all he will understand is the simple pleasure of being able to move his bowels. Neither he nor his wife will ever understand the hell I went through to put him on that toilet. Like Mr. Baker, most patients will never know what their surgeon had to go through to get them safely off the operating room table and out of the hospital. Most patients will never know because *most will recover without complications.*

Even good surgeons can get into trouble during an operation. Anything can happen, at any time, to the best of us. A good surgeon must be able to recognize trouble, get out of it, and avoid or minimize any subsequent damage to the patient. This is one of the essential qualities that defines a good surgeon. The problem is, patients can't find this qualification in any curriculum vitae or on any credentialing list. There is no wall diploma documenting this particular ability, no data available on how often your surgeon has experienced complications or how well they were corrected. I recommend that you ask your surgeon how often he or she has experienced a major complication specific to your upcoming operation.

I know I can get in (and out) of trouble. I have had my share of mishaps in the operating room, most of which I was able to correct without causing permanent harm. Every single day, my goal is the same: Avoid getting into trouble in the first place; avoid the stress of having to deal with it. This is a more difficult goal when starting out in practice. When you are a new surgeon, you can't draw on past experiences when facing unexpected trouble in the operating room because you just do not have them. Over the last twenty years, I have experienced every known complication specific to my specialty inside the operating room. The one thing I haven't done is operate on the wrong body part. Not yet, anyway.

There is an old saying passed down among surgeons that still rings true today: The first ten years of practice, a surgeon learns *how* to operate. When I finished training, I wasn't comfortable with my skills inside the operating room. I was considered a safe surgeon, but some operations scared the living daylights out of me. Operations on the pancreas or the upper parts of the stomach fell into this category. These were scary because I just didn't have enough experience performing them. Experience leads to familiarity and self-confidence, both essential to good judgment in the operating room. Experience should lead to wisdom, and wisdom includes acknowledging my limitations.

It takes time and experience to perfect techniques and build confidence. How much time? It varies, just like every surgeon's ability. Some surgeons need only months, some need years, and yet others are still developing these skills well into their careers. During the first ten years of my practice, I was eager to operate on anyone who walked into my office and needed an operation. I was fresh out of residency and champing at the bit to get into the operating room. I was eager to show off my stuff, build a practice, and make some money. Who wouldn't be after eight years of school and five years of training, making what (if you calculated the hours) amounted to third-world wages?

The second part of the old adage states: The second ten years of practice, a surgeon learns *when* to operate. After a period of years operating, most surgeons (those with a conscience, anyway) start to get a little selective about whom they choose to take to the operating room. With certain diseases, the indication for an elective operation can be a wide gray zone, left up to the honest, good judgment of your surgeon. This is why you can go to two different surgeons and get two different opinions. Ideally, as surgeons gain experience, they continue to fine-tune their surgical judgment. The timing of an operation on a critically ill patient can mean the difference between life and death. There are patients I have waited on too long, hoping their illness might improve. There are also some for whom I have pulled out the scalpel too soon. Some of these patients have lived and some have died. Of the ones that died, some would have anyway regardless of what I decided to do. Each one taught me an invaluable lesson that I carried into the second ten years of my practice.

And finally: The last ten years of practice, a surgeon learns when *not* to operate. I believe this is the most important and most difficult lesson any surgeon can learn. It's the most important because a surgeon's knife can not only save a life; it can end one as well. As my career has progressed, experience has helped me determine when *not* to take someone to the operating room. The fact is, many of the ill patients that I am asked to evaluate will get better with *nonsurgical* remedies. And some are just too sick to see the inside of the operating room. In these situations, I often have to resist my basic cutting instincts, be realistic with families, and rely on lessons learned from past experiences. I have to resist my urge to "do something" and squelch the fear of waiting too long. This is very difficult to do. I am a surgeon, and to cut is to cure. It takes discipline and seasoned judgment (based on years of experience) to forgo the knife and allow other medical treatments to work.

In every surgeon's career, there are operations that not only test our physical skills and judgment but also challenge the very core of what we are made of. My test arrived in the form of Mr. John Jacobs. Mr. Jacobs was a seventy-nine-year-old gentleman with a history of worsening Parkinson's disease. He had been in the hospital for several days with abdominal pain from gallstones before I was asked to see him. Despite being treated with antibiotics, he continued to have pain and fevers along with a rising white blood cell count. Every test pointed to a serious infection in his gallbladder that only an operation would cure. I took one look at this shrunken, frail, sick soul lying in his intensive care bed and knew surgery would be very risky for him. If I did operate, the risk of a serious complication during surgery was high. I suspected his gallbladder would be an inflamed mess and would not succumb without a fight. The last thing I wanted was to add to this man's misery—if he survived—by making a serious mistake during the surgery.

"Jackie," I turned to his nurse, "I do not want to operate on this guy. Surgery will be too much of a stress for him." Not a word from Jackie. "I don't want to put the last nail in his coffin." I spoke softly but Mr. Jacobs was too sick to understand anything anyway. "Hell, what choice do I have," I continued, thinking out loud. "If I don't operate he most assuredly will die from sepsis. His only chance is surgery and prayer. The family wants everything done so I'll give them everything." I was looking for someone, anyone to talk me out of it. I was trying to talk myself out of it. Jackie wasn't helping. I was having another of those conversations surgeons have with themselves. No one was going to help me with this decision or the many others soon to follow. This was mine to make and mine to live with.

"Jackie, I don't want this man dying on the table on me." She looked at me, silent.

The last thing any surgeon wants is to lose a patient on the operating room table. We will do whatever it takes to get someone through an operation and off the table alive. I consider it a momentous failure and personal loss when I lose someone in the operating room. I am a surgeon. I am all-powerful. I can do anything, save everyone. How dare you die under my knife? No one is allowed to die when I am operating. It is almost as if my anger is directed at the patient for dying on me. And anger is one of the emotions I feel when this happens. I am angry because death, to me, means I have failed in the eyes of a family who relied on my judgment. It means I have failed my own expectations. It means I failed somewhere along the decision process. Maybe I should have acted sooner? I am also angry because months later I will have to relive my failure in front of my peers at our monthly department of surgery meeting. And later, I may have to relive my failure in a courtroom. As a surgeon, I have difficulty facing failure. We are trained not to accept failure.

Losing a patient on the operating room table also forces me to face another uncomfortable aspect of my job. It is humbling to walk into a waiting room full of anxious family members who are desperately hoping for some good news, and deliver an announcement of death. How to deliver bad news is not taught in medical school or residency. As with operating, though, surgeons get better at this with experience. Being the bearer of bad news is something I don't want to get good at.

As I thought about how I would prepare the family for the potential consequences of the operation, my hand reached down to touch Mr. Jacobs's upper abdomen. He recoiled in pain. "Peritonitis." My response was automatic. "My decision is made. Call the operating room."

I had been introduced to Mr. Jacobs's family by his primary care doctor as the "best" surgeon to do the job, the best man to take care of their beloved father. It wasn't my idea of a good introduction because it could give the family false hope and raise their expectations too high.

My instincts were correct about Mr. Jacobs. After I opened him up, his diseased gallbladder proved to be one of the worst I had ever encountered. It was angry. I was angry because of what I knew was to come.

How in the world am I going to get this thing out without damaging something? Another conversation with another diseased organ. *Just look at what I have to work with!* As the surgery progressed, my eye caught a wisp of a yellow liquid coming from underneath his liver. It stopped me in my tracks.

"Nurse, what the hell is that?" I knew very well what it was but was not ready to face it. "Where is that coming from?" Again, I knew the answer but was terrified of even saying the words. "Son of a bitch." I had to step back to regain my composure. I could feel my legs shaking and my anal sphincter losing its muscle tone. It was a bile leak. As I was removing the gallbladder from the underside of the liver, I accidentally cut across the common bile duct. The common bile duct is a long, thin tube that delivers bile from the liver into the intestine. The gallbladder is an offshoot of this tube.

I fucking cut across his common bile duct. I felt like passing out. Injuring the common bile duct during gallbladder surgery is *the* most feared complication any general surgeon can experience. It is the nuclear bomb of general surgery complications. When it occurs, it is physically devastating for the patient and mentally destabilizing for the surgeon. Throughout the years, I'd had some close calls on several occasions. Even the close calls give a surgeon with a conscience fits inside the operating room, and insomnia at home. But I thought *this*—a severed bile duct— would never happen to me. With this type of complication in this setting, the best I could do was to divert the leaking bile out of the abdomen with a drain and complete the removal of the gallbladder. This was a temporary Band-Aid. The injury itself was a much more serious problem that would need further surgery to correct, surgery I was not comfortable performing. My thought was to get him off the table and transferred to a teaching center for further care. Even if the additional surgery is successful, patients who experience this type of injury are seldom ever the same.

As I placated my mistake, random thoughts circulated through my head. I thought about this patient's slow demise as his family watched; admitting my mistake; explaining my complication to his internist, who trusted me; an early retirement; and even entering the priesthood. (I have a brother who is a priest and I could have used his blessing before my first cut.) My hands continued to operate on Mr. Jacobs, but my mind was racing. *Now I really did it. I probably killed this guy. What am I going to tell the family? I might as well just have my malpractice company write the check out now. Why wait?* I was exhausted, panicking, and not making much sense. The worst part was I had no idea I had cut through the bile duct when I did. I just went right through that stop sign. The only saving grace was that I recognized the injury soon after it was made and did what I could to minimize the damage, if only temporarily.

The entire Jacobs family was in the waiting room, waiting for the good news from the best surgeon about their dad's operation. It was a large family. I did not have good news for them today. I was beaten down, knowing I soon would have to explain my mistake to an audience. I should have been satisfied the man survived the surgery and was on his way to the intensive care unit. Satisfaction was the furthest thing from my mind. My hands were shaking.

As I approached the room, my mind reviewed various explanations I could offer up for my mishap. Maybe I could push the blame away—to Mr. Jacobs's severely diseased gallbladder, or the internist who called me into this mess, or the full moon that night. I wanted to blame anything but myself. This was my first instinct, an instinct born out of survival. What I do is not an exact science; mistakes happen. When mistakes do happen, patients suffer and surgeons get punished mentally, physically, and financially. I needed some excuse to offer up to the family and buffer the shock. There wasn't one. I was solely to blame. I was tired, upset, humbled, and alone. All I wanted was to crawl into an empty hospital bed, pull the covers over my head, and not be a surgeon anymore.

In a recent survey of American surgeons, 9 percent reported they had made a *major* medical error in the last three months. As I approached Mr. Jacobs's family in the waiting room, I became part of that 9 percent.

"Mrs. Jacobs." I approached her slowly. There must have been at least ten family members hovering around her. They all stood up. I took her right hand and looked in her eyes. I wanted her to see my face. "Your husband is fine. His gallbladder was badly diseased. He did well throughout the operation despite being so sick."

"Oh, thank you so much, Dr. Ruggieri!" I had to stop her in midsentence.

"But, Mrs. Jacobs"—I swallowed hard—"as I was removing his gallbladder, I inadvertently cut his main bile duct." A collective gasp came from the rest of the family. Shock was evident on their faces. I had not prepared the family well enough in advance for this news. Hell, I had not prepared myself to deliver it.

As a surgeon about to operate on someone critically ill, I am responsible for preparing the family before I enter the operating room for the potential of a bad outcome. This is a crucial task for any surgeon; it will lessen the blow of a complication or death after an operation. Anticipating the worst is another survival tool all surgeons must know how to apply effectively. In emergency situations, before I open a patient up, I generally know what I might find and how sick that person will be afterward. If I don't plant a realistic seed when preparing family members for all possibilities, I do them an injustice. I also put myself at risk. Family members do not like surprises, especially when it arrives in the form of a complication or death. A number of times during my career, a patient's clinical presentation has led me to anticipate the worst. For these critically ill patients, I do what I have been trained to do to get them through surgery and give them a realistic chance of survival. In these situations, a surgeon's work starts well before the first cut is made.

With Mrs. Jacobs, I had to tell her the painful truth about what had happened. "It was my fault and I am sorry." I just wanted to die. After regaining some semblance of composure, I proceeded to explain to her why something like this could happen and the long-term consequences. I also explained my plan

(I had to have a plan) to provide Mr. Jacobs with the best care. I am not sure how much sank in after the initial shock, but in the end, Mr. Jacobs was transferred to a major medical center in the area for further treatment. I limped home under the cover of early-morning darkness. Another day was soon to arrive.

In my work as a surgeon, the operating room is my kingdom, my sanctuary from the stresses of the rest of the hospital and the outside world. As Tessio, in the original *Godfather* movie, once said, "This is my territory. I rule it." It is a secretive place where I can keep myself secluded for hours, protected from any outside demands. If the nurses on the floor have questions about my other patients and I don't feel like answering, my standard answer is, "I can't deal with this right now. I'm operating." If the emergency room is calling me to see a patient, my answer can be, "I can't deal with this now. I'm operating." If my wife wants me and I don't feel like talking, "I'm operating." If my malpractice lawyer is calling to set up a deposition date on a case I was involved with, "I am operating all month, and then on vacation." The operating room is a sacred place, where I rule and have sovereign power. I decide who comes in and who leaves. I decide what instruments to use. Ultimately, it is largely my skills and judgment that will determine what shape a patient is in when he or she leaves the room.

To most patients, the operating room is a mysterious and intimidating place. (How can it not be, knowing that one doctor is going to put you to sleep so that another one can cut you open?) The anesthesiologist is the most important player with your surgeon during an operation. The job of the anesthesiologist is quite basic: He or she keeps you physiologically alive during surgery. The anesthesiologist is in constant communication with your surgeon, looking to anticipate and prevent problems before they arise. While your surgeon is removing or repairing organs, the anesthesiologist is breathing for you, constantly monitoring vital body functions. As important as it is for you to know how competent your surgeon is, it is as important or *more* important to know who your anesthesiologist is. Like surgeons, anesthesiologists come in all shapes, sizes, and skill sets. Unlike surgeons, anesthesiologists don't have an office in the community. They work at hospitals, within the secluded walls of the operating room. Their reputations are hard to track down and difficult to evaluate. Their track record is generally not exposed for all to see and judge. My advice: Ask your surgeon which anesthesiologist he or she recommends; then, request a consultation with the anesthesiologist. Go with a list of questions (ask your surgeon if you don't know what to ask). Some hospitals will make this difficult, but you can insist on it.

As a surgical patient, you hand over control of your body, temporarily bestowing total trust on the surgeon holding the knife and the anesthesiologist wielding the dream drugs. The surrender continues as you move, half-naked with your butt hanging out, to a cold stainless steel operating room table seemingly the width of a Hershey's bar. Quickly, the fear of falling onto the floor turns to claustrophobia as the anesthesiologist places the oxygen mask over your face. (I often get claustrophobic just watching that mask descend upon my patients.) Once asleep, you have no idea what is being done to you. The submission finally ends when you wake up, desperately trying to cough life back into your lungs. Every day, I am awed by patients as they trust their limbs, organs, and lives to me, hoping they will leave the operating room in better shape than when they entered. Every day, most do.

As a general surgeon working within the operating room, I have seen it all. I have been involved in operations that have been perfect, and others that have gone horribly wrong. I have seen the extremes of what those in my profession can do during the most stressful times in an operating room. I have seen the best and the worst of personal and professional behaviors under high-pressure situations. The doings of the operating room can wreak havoc on a surgeon's psyche and ego. It is a place of both great triumphs and unexpected tragedies. It is a place where lives are saved and lives (and limbs and organs) are lost. It is a place where surgeons can experience a plethora of emotions during a single operation. In the span of two short hours, the operating room can go from boring to terrifying, from exciting to devastating. One minute I can be in the middle of a perfect dissection; the next, in a cold sweat with my heart racing as blood wells up from something I have accidentally disturbed. For a patient, the operating room can be a frightening place. For surgeons, it is so much more.

Chapter 6

///

Surgeons Hate Surprises

"Dr. Ruggieri, please come to the emergency room stat." I was in the middle of slicing through a buttock abscess the size of a tangerine on a young man when the overhead page spoke out.

"Damn, Doc, that hurts." I smiled, ignoring his cries. The man let out a short howl. "I thought you were going to numb it."

Be quiet, will you! I strained to hear the page. *Suck it up. It'll be over in a minute.* I had anesthetized the area, but knew the procedure would still be painful. ("You may experience some discomfort," is how most surgeons like to frame it for patients.) My job involves inflicting pain. I am a surgeon. And now I was in a hurry. "I think they need me in the emergency room," I told him. The pus was flowing like lava spewing out of a volcano. I was hurrying it along with my fingers.

"Just got to love this," I mumbled. I paused briefly to admire my work and turned my head to take a deep breath of fresh air away from the odor. Draining pus is what general surgeons do best and do often. The procedure is not glamorous. It requires no thinking. Anyone with two working digits, one good eye, and a sharp knife can do it. It is simple and fast, and the outcome is predictable. There are no surprises here. No sleepless nights worrying. No long explanations on what to expect. It is a procedure that's impossible to screw up and one that leaves patients pleased.

A second page rang out from the ceiling speaker. "Dr. Ruggieri, you are needed in the emergency room *now*."

"Doc, this still hurts." The young man was squirming. I pretended to listen to him.

"Okay. I need to go. Nurse, can you pack this for me? Have him see me in the office next week." I placed her hand on the gauze covering the oozing abscess.

By the time I entered the main trauma room in the E.R., the paramedics were already well into a round of C.P.R. The crack, crack, crack of broken ribs with each chest compression greeted me at the door. The death clock had started.

"Guys, easy on the ribs. If he lives you'll have some explaining to do." I got closer. "Who is this?" I glanced at the patient on the table. My heart rate began to increase. I had to look away then, and steel myself. It was a little boy at the end of those chest compressions and cracked ribs. A little boy with blond hair. I couldn't let my stirred-up emotions from seeing a child near death interfere with the decisions ahead. *I* have *to do this; otherwise I am no use to anyone.* An emotional heart is not welcome inside a trauma or operating room. It has to be left at the door. A surgeon can't afford any distractions at a time like this.

"Hold compressions." The monitor was a flat line, asystolic. No heart activity, no life. "Keep pumping. Go, man, go!" The seconds continued to slip away. I glanced at his partially covered face, blue eyes wide open. Another paramedic was trying to keep his lungs full of oxygen through a breathing tube. The compressions continued. "Does anyone know what happened here?" More cracking. I was looking for something, any clue as to why this patient arrived in my emergency room clinically dead.

"All we know, Doc, is it was some accident at home with a knife. It was found in another room with blood on it." The paramedic continued, "When we arrived, he was on the kitchen floor alone, no heartbeat, and white as a ghost." More seconds lost. "I didn't see any parents. One of the neighbors said his name is Jason." More seconds were lost. More brain cells were dying. I did not have much time to figure this out.

"Get the rest of his clothes off now." I ran through the list of the different causes of asystole in my head, seeing if any would apply to Jason. With his clothes off, I was able to inspect every inch of this little blond patient. "He must not even be ten years old." I had to work hard to keep my heart out of the room. Upon initial survey of his skinny little body, peppered with freckles, nothing was obvious.

"What the hell happened here?" I was shouting at the heart monitor.

"Doc, no blood pressure. We are losing him." Sweat was dripping down the paramedic's temple.

"Keep pumping." I looked at his lifeless eyes for a clue as to what had happened. I wanted to shake him. "Wake up, boy. Help me here. Tell me what happened so I can do something to keep you alive!" My heart was racing and his heart was dying. I scanned his naked body again in desperation.

"Wait, stop compressions for a second." I motioned to the paramedic. "Move your hand away from his chest." There it was at the base of his sternum, the clue to bringing this boy back. I hadn't seen it at first because the chest compressions had covered it. There was no time to gloat, no time to pat myself on the back. The boy had only one chance and it was slim, at best. "Look at that, see it?" I pointed to a half inch break of skin just below his breastbone. "Son of a bitch. See that entrance wound. He's in cardiac tamponade. Was the kid playing with a knife?" All I saw were blank faces. A knife somehow must have sneaked underneath his breastbone, piercing his heart. The hole caused blood to escape the heart chamber and immediately fill the sac surrounding it. Pressure from the accumulating blood squeezes the heart, giving it no room to pump. The heart suffocates under the weight of its own blood. If nothing is done to relieve the pressure, life is over quickly.

"Nurse, open the thoracotomy tray." It was time to move.

Immediately, my training instincts took over. I had to slice open this boy's chest and gain access to his heart. His only chance at survival was for me to remove the blood surrounding his heart, stop the leak, and jump start the heart back to life. All emergency rooms have thoracotomy trays in them for just this reason. The operation to access the heart in this setting is called a thoracotomy (cutting into the thorax or chest cavity). Thoracotomy trays contain the instruments, bundled together, necessary for the operation.

An emergency thoracotomy is an operation of last resort. It is a procedure often performed out of heroic desperation on patients with penetrating injuries to the heart. In certain rare situations when a heart injury is recognized early enough, it can save lives—*if* performed before irreversible heart damage has occurred. The reality is that most patients die before ever making it to the emergency room. For the ones who do make it to the hospital, the procedure often ends up being a mini-autopsy, or a teaching experience.

Despite its dismal success, any surgical resident in training is eager to get the opportunity to perform an emergency thoracotomy because it means membership in an elite club. If, by the grace of God, the patient lives, you will forever go down in surgical lore. Among surgical brethren, the procedure is considered the most macho of them all. It is filled with a mix of fear, adrenaline, and testosterone. Just imagine having the power to slice open the chest of a patient at death's door, blood flying, suturing the hole, and shocking a dead heart back to life. Talk about a rush. Early in my career, this is what I lived for. I lived for the unexpected opportunity to stare death in the face and say, *Take that! Not on my watch.* Even if the thoracotomy fails, what is there to lose? The patient is already dead. I was fortunate to have performed one of these procedures as a surgical resident on a patient stabbed in the chest. It wasn't the best of techniques, but the experience served its teaching purpose at the time. That patient left the trauma room dead, in a body bag. I left the trauma room alive, and a hero.

"Shock him one last time before I go in." Still flatline. "Nurse, hand me a knife. Everyone, move your hands away." The adrenaline was flowing. I splashed some antiseptic on his left chest and started my cut at the middle of his breastbone. *Keep your hand steady and just cut.* It was a deep cut, circling underneath his left nipple and angling toward his armpit. Despite the shaking, I managed to go through skin, fat, and muscle in one deep slice. The hardness of his ribs was the only thing that stopped me from cutting right into his lung. I was happy with that. *Like cutting through butter,* I thought to myself. I accidentally nicked his nipple on the way up. *Shit. Sorry. Can't worry about it now.* There wasn't much bleeding. "This is not good. Nurse, hand me the scissors." I was sweating profusely. In one sweeping motion, I cut through the muscles connecting the ribs below his nipple and the lining of lung beneath. "There it is. Jackpot. Nurse, rib spreader." More cracking. Young ribs separate with little effort. I frantically sucked out the clumps of blood suffocating the boy's heart.

"Doc, there's the hole." The paramedic doing the chest compressions was completely exhausted.

"I see it." I took a needle the size of a large fishhook and blindly placed two sutures on each side of my finger plugging the hole. "Nurse, please don't let me stick myself." Blood was everywhere. The sutures were tied and it worked. The hole was closed.

"Charge the paddles," I bellowed. The hole was closed but the heart was dead. Electricity was the only way to bring it back.

"Clear!" I cupped Jason's flaccid heart in the defibrillator paddles. "Hit it!" I loved saying this with life in the balance. The moment brought me as close to playing God as I will ever get. The boy's back arched up off the table. Still flatline. "Increase the voltage. Again, hit it." Another arch, another shock, and more flatline.

"Doc, what's that odor?" The paramedic looked at the burn marks left by the paddles on the boy's chest. "Sorry, Doc. I should have used more gel."

This cycle of electrical shock, arching back, flatline, and chest compressions went on for another thirty minutes. For a few seconds, Jason's heart would quiver after a jolt, teasing us into thinking there was hope of bringing him back. There wasn't. The ten-year-old boy on the table had died on his kitchen floor from a knife wound piercing his heart.

After I called it off, everyone left the room without saying a word. Everyone, except me. It was my job to make the boy whole again. Since I was the one who opened up his chest, I was the one to suture it back together. I had to make Jason presentable to his grieving parents. My hands moved quickly to suture his ribs closed. The broken ones would not come together quietly. The adrenaline rush from making life-and-death decisions was over, replaced by the empty reality of a young death. I had nowhere to hide. While I sutured, my mind became preoccupied with doubt. *Could I have recognized the knife wound sooner? Did I act in time? What else could have I done differently?* When the unexpected arrives unannounced and exits with a bad outcome, I am always revisiting my actions.

"Doc." A policeman walked in, his voice interrupting one of

my sutures. "We have preliminary evidence the boy's death was no accident."

"What do you mean?" I continued to suture. The dead muscle would be next, followed by fat and skin.

"There was a witness." I could see that the policeman was struggling with the sight of an open chest on a dead ten-year-old boy. "The boy's father and mother were fighting." He put his hand to his mouth. "The father grabbed a kitchen knife." He looked away. "The boy was just trying to help his mom. It all happened so fast."

"Thanks for the information." I just shook my head. The policeman stumbled out. I struggled to pull all the sutures together tightly, closing the gap between the boy's ribs. Jason was whole again. Suddenly, my pager went off. The guy with the buttock abscess was bleeding through his bandages.

That was predictable. This, I can live with. On the way out, I stopped at the door and checked back in with my own heart. It was still beating.

///

One of the most consistent aspects of my job is its unpredictability. From the first day of training, there has been a never-ending line of patient experiences that can be categorized as befuddling, frightening, exhilarating, and unapologetically shocking. As a surgical resident, I relished every one of these experiences because each one presented an opportunity to learn, to gain experience in diagnosing and treating the most unexpected surgical illnesses. More important, these cases presented opportunities to get inside the operating room. Most of these experiences came to me via the E.R., the emergency room.

I was three weeks into my training when I was introduced to Mr. Jackson. He walked in off the street with a simple laceration to his arm, checked in at the E.R. desk, and was placed on an emergency room bed. I soon followed him into the room.

"Doc, I was doing some work in my backyard when I accidentally cut myself," he said nonchalantly. The explanation seemed likely enough.

"Let's take a look." It wasn't a big laceration, but he was a big guy. "I'll have you out of here in no time. I need to get some supplies." I walked out the door, heading for some suture material when two policemen started to come at me. They motioned for me to duck into an adjacent room.

"Doc, the guy you just saw is wanted in a murder investigation. His name came across our system when he checked into the emergency room." They were serious. I just wanted to suture up a laceration.

"Okay." I took a deep breath and pointed to the suture material on the table. "You go sew him up because I am not going back in there. Suturing up murder suspects is not in my job description. I have enough to do already."

"Doc, you need to go back in there. Act like you don't know anything." They weren't kidding.

"Guys, I'm an intern. I'm not supposed to know anything." They smiled. I was petrified.

"Doc, when you are finished suturing him up, just act normal and leave the room. We'll take it from there."

Before going back, I turned my badge around to hide my name. Without saying much, I nervously sutured Mr. Jackson's laceration and bandaged his arm. "Mr. Jackson, come and see me in the clinic in a week to remove the sutures."

"No problem, Doc." He started to get dressed.

I quickly grabbed anything sharp I had brought into the room and walked out. I managed to duck into an adjacent men's room, closing the door behind me. Mr. Jackson exited the room soon after, walking right into the arms of two very large city policemen. I made sure he was out of the building before resuming my duties.

Over the next six weeks in the emergency room, I was introduced to a variety of individuals, several billed as "You need to see this to believe it!" Phillip was one such case. He was a local construction worker, working on a job downtown. He had been involved in an accident on the job and brought to the emergency room for treatment. The dispatcher did not mince words: "Bringing in a thirty-five-year-old male, construction worker, with a rod impaled in his chest." I thought, *Why couldn't he wait another hour, when my shift is up? How in the world am I going to manage this? The guy is probably going to bleed to death as soon as he gets here. Why me?*

I could hear the ambulance sirens in the distance getting closer and closer.

"Waiting for these trauma patients to arrive drives me nuts." I was pacing in the main trauma room, trying to calm myself down by talking to one of the nurses. "You never know what the hell you are going to get when the paramedics drop off their loot." I was searching for scissors to cut his clothes off as soon as he arrived. "The sirens are getting louder. They are almost here. Let's go." I ran out to meet the stretcher to get an up-close look at the damage. The ambulance door opened and a man with a steel rod coming out of his chest greeted me.

"Doc"—Phillip was awake and coherent—"sorry. I slipped and fell two floors down onto some steel rods. My wife is going to kill me. We had plans to have friends over to the house tonight." He grimaced at the rod rooted in his chest. "I feel like a Popsicle. Doc, it hurts when I breathe."

"I *bet* it hurts." I could only laugh in amazement. The guy was awake and conversing with three feet of quarter-inch steel rebar sticking out of the middle of his chest. Phillip had impaled himself on the rod during his fall. His coworkers had quickly freed him up by cutting through the lower end with their welding torches.

"Man, you are one lucky son of a bitch. This thing must have had eyes going in." His vital signs were remarkably stable. "What the hell am I going to do with this rod?"

"Doc, get it out of there." The rod moved slightly with each deep breath.

Somehow, the rod had managed to sneak its way around all the major organs in Phillip's chest cavity. One millionth of an inch in either direction would have meant instant death.

"I'm not touching this thing here. We need to get you to the operating room." I quickly surveyed his body for any other injuries.

"Doc, I don't care where you do it. Just get it out so I can get home." I made some phone calls. Within minutes, Phillip was whisked upstairs to a waiting operating room. Once he was under anesthesia, I opened Phillip's left chest to gain access to the rod as it disappeared into his left lung. I had to gain proximal and distal control of any major vessels pierced by the rod before inching it out or he would bleed to death on the table. From what I could see, all the important blood vessels were missed. The heart was untouched as well. It appeared that the lung had taken the brunt of the impalement. Once I convinced myself that nothing major was compromised, the rest was easy. The rod was removed and any bleeding from the damaged lung was easy to contain. Phillip recovered very well, suffering no permanent injuries and returning to work one month later.

///

A week after I met Phillip, a middle-aged man arrived at the emergency room after being gorged in the leg by a rhinoceros at the local zoo. He had been a little too curious on his visit to the rhino exhibit, falling over the rail into the rhino's lair. The rhino was not happy to find an intruder in his yard, so he attacked him with his horn. The patient was brought in as having sustained "a stable laceration to his right thigh with a lot of blood at the scene." When he arrived, I slowly cut through the bandages to look at the injury. "What is your name?" I asked, trying to distract his attention from what I was doing.

"Larry." He was trying not to look at his leg.

"Larry, you pissed off a rhinoceros at the zoo today. You will be fine, but we are going to have to take you to the operating room to clean this out." I slowly peeled back the blood-soaked bandages. "Duck!" I yelled out. A pulsing stream of blood instantly jetted out, grazing my left temple and nailing the wall behind me. "Stable laceration, my ass. This man has a major femoral artery injury. Get him ready to go to the operating room *now*!" I hate surprises, especially bloody ones.

///

Dr. Stiller was a pathologist at the local hospital. He was also a colleague and a good friend. I was honored that he had chosen me to perform his surgery. (It is always good for the ego when a colleague chooses me to perform surgery.) He arrived in my office after experiencing a syndrome of intermittent pain in his upper abdomen after meals. X-ray studies indicated that he had gallstones. Dr. Stiller's symptoms fit the classic pain description for gallstones, so it was obvious what needed to be done next. It all seemed too easy, especially because Dr. Stiller was a thin man with no risk factors for complications. Here was a case where classic symptoms of pain had led to predictable imaging studies diagnosing gallstones, which led to a simple solution: surgery.

I love gallstones because the diagnosis is usually obvious and patients are very satisfied after surgery. Laparoscopic cholecystectomy is one of the most common operations performed in this country. It involves removing the gallbladder through very small incisions. It is a quick, boring operation with few surprises.

Inside the operating room, Dr. Stiller's operation was progressing routinely, like the hundreds I had performed before his.

But before removing the gallbladder, I decided to inject x-ray dye into the common bile duct, which is attached to the gallbladder. The subsequent x-ray is called a cholangiogram. I do it to see if any stones have leaked into the common bile duct. If stones are present, they will need to be removed at a later date, by a different procedure. It was a last-minute decision, partly because it was easy to do and partly because I was paranoid about missing something. In surgery, Murphy's Law seems to kick in when operating on fellow doctors, doctors' wives, nurses, lawyers, lawyers' wives, or any other high-profile patients. Be assured: If anything can go wrong, it will!

Often, surgeons bypass the cholangiogram if there is no suspicion before surgery (based on blood tests) that stones exist in the main duct. As I waited for the dye to outline the long, smooth pipelike contour of Dr. Stiller's common bile duct, I was already getting stressed about the next operation. The patient was a forty-five-year-old woman who needed her thyroid gland removed because of a cancerous nodule. She had a fat neck and loved to sing in her church's choir. Fat necks make removing someone's thyroid gland difficult, and thyroid surgery (in the wrong hands) can be hazardous to one's voice. The main complication of thyroid surgery is injury to the nerves that control movement of the vocal cords. These nerves run right up against the thyroid gland and have to be *gently* moved out of the way. This is, literally, a nerve-racking part of the operation, contributing to the gray hairs on my head. If I injure these nerves—in any way—my patient's singing career is over, my thyroid surgery practice takes a hit, and my malpractice insurance premiums rise.

"Doc, is that picture good enough?" The x-ray technician's voice brought me back to Dr. Stiller's operation.

"What is that down there?" I pointed to the irregular narrowing at the tapered end of the bile duct. "See that? It doesn't look right. This outline should be much smoother." I stared at the picture for a few seconds. *This can't be. Don't even think about it.* I had seen this narrowing before, mostly after someone has passed a gallstone. It is often nothing to worry about, but it needs to be worked up after the surgery.

"There is nothing to do about this now. I'll get one of the G. I. docs to take a look up there in several weeks. Let's get this gallbladder out and get him off the table." I did not want any more surprises.

After Dr. Stiller fully recovered from his surgery, I had him follow up with a gastroenterologist for a procedure called endoscopic retrograde cholangiopancreatography (E.R.C.P.). The doctor places a long, thin scope into the main common bile duct by going through the stomach and can look directly into the duct to see what is inside.

Several months later, I received a call from the gastroenterologist who had performed the E.R.C.P. on Dr. Stiller. "He has a cancer of the main bile duct."

"What?" I had to sit down.

"The narrowing you incidentally discovered on the x-ray is a bile duct cancer. The biopsies came back positive." I could hear the pessimism in the gastroenterologist's voice.

"I can't believe it. I almost didn't shoot the x-ray during his surgery. I would have missed this thing entirely." On another day, I might have elected not to shoot the x-ray, probably delaying for months the diagnosis of cancer in my colleague.

Bile duct cancer is one of the deadliest cancers diagnosed today. The symptoms are subtle and insidious and often go unnoticed early in the disease. They can range from a mild, intermittent upper abdominal pain to weight loss. By the time the cancer is diagnosed, it has often spread to other parts of the body and is incurable. If, by a stroke of luck, it is diagnosed early, the only curable chance a patient has is surgery. The survival rate for bile duct cancer is dismal, even for those who have been diagnosed early. For those who have had curative surgery, the five-year survival rate is 20 to 40 percent. For patients with metastasis at the time of diagnosis, most will succumb to the disease within a year.

Dr. Stiller went on to have a major, curative operation to remove his bile duct cancer. Fortunately, for him, the cancer was in an early stage and effectively treated with surgery. Despite the good outcome, there are days when I wonder how often I have missed or delayed the opportunity to diagnose something unexpected, something potentially curable.

///

To me, *routine* is a beautiful word.

I really do hate surprises inside (and outside) the operating room. In the operating room, I am somewhat of a control freak. I want to be in a position where I know exactly what I am getting into before I get into it. I want to control the tempo of any situation and minimize the influence of the unknown. I want to be in total control of events during an operation, relying, if possible, only on myself. This is one of the reasons I became a surgeon. I wanted the ability to diagnose a tangible illness, treat it with a tangible operation, and immediately obtain tangible results. I wanted to rely solely on my trained abilities to achieve specific outcomes.

As a surgeon, I can diagnose a physical illness and treat it with something physical, a knife. If an organ needs to be removed, I want to remove it. If something needs to be drained, I want to drain it. If something needs to be repaired, I want to repair it. I do not want to sit back and rely on drugs to treat something I cannot touch, see, or smell.

I despise the unknown. The last thing I want is to be surprised by something in the operating room. Surprises mean added stress, longer procedures, inadequate operations, messed-up schedules, the potential for complications, and the possibility of unexpected outcomes. Surprises mean I was off with my diagnosis. Surprises mean I may have missed something subtle and was not totally prepared for the operation. I view surprises as a reflection of my imperfection, a reflection of not being able to accurately judge a situation.

Patients and families are not fond of surprises either. Surprises mean longer explanations to family members after an operation. They also generate questions. *Doctor, why didn't that show up on the blood work or the x-ray? Doctor, why didn't you suspect that before going in? Doctor, what does this mean?* It can be difficult to explain an unexpected finding at the time of an operation without stepping on my own confidence.

Despite wanting to know exactly what I am dealing with *before* my knife hits the skin, there are times when I've done all the tests allowed by insurance companies and yet *still* have no diagnosis. There are times when I don't have a surgical answer to a patient's complaints. There are times I can't give a patient the comfort of a confident diagnosis without an operation.

An exploratory laparotomy is one of the most common operations I perform as a general surgeon. The words literally mean to *explore the abdomen*. It is an operation performed as the final test to arrive at a diagnosis. It is performed on patients with abdominal complaints whose test results suggest something abnormal inside their abdomen. What that something is often can only be determined by a major surgical exploration of the abdominal cavity. Today, that major surgery is performed in two ways. The first: using a long abdominal incision and my hands. The second: using very small incisions, a camera (laparoscope), and tiny instruments. Either method can be effective depending on the indication for surgery, the patient's body contour, history of previous abdominal surgery, underlying medical problems— and the surgeon's skill.

In emergency situations, an exploratory laparotomy is performed to stop life-threatening internal bleeding from an ulcer, colon disease, or injured spleen. Whatever the reason may be, I am not happy when forced to take someone back to the operating room to stop bleeding of which I was the cause. Postoperative internal bleeding after major abdominal surgery is an event no surgeon expects but must face on occasion. In some situations, the bleeding stops spontaneously. Patients may require transfusions, but repeat surgery is often avoided. Internal hemorrhaging after surgery gives me nightmares. These are tenuous situations because the timing of the decision to reoperate is crucial. If I reoperate too soon, the stress of another immediate surgery may be fatal. If I wait too long, the delay may be fatal.

I consider it a professional failure if I have to reexplore a patient for bleeding immediately after major surgery. It is difficult to face on a professional level because of the potential patient harm it can lead to. On a personal level, having to reexplore a patient for bleeding that I caused indirectly is humbling, embarrassing, and upsetting. When it occurs, I consider it a failure of my surgical skills and judgment. It is also unexpected and frightening news for a patient's family. Having to explain to a patient and family the need for an emergent reoperation to stop internal bleeding is not an enviable position to be in.

The reoperation rate for bleeding after any surgery is a true benchmark of a surgeon's skills and judgment inside the operating room. When a surgeon's reoperation rates are not in line with those of his or her colleagues, it may indicate problems. Every hospital has information on its surgeons' reoperation rates for bleeding. Like other measures of a surgeon's abilities, this information is not for your eyes. Every surgeon is keenly aware of his or her own reoperative rates for bleeding. I know mine. Do you know your surgeon's?

Mr. John Flint walked into my office because he needed an exploratory laparotomy. He wasn't bleeding. He was not acutely ill. He just hadn't been feeling right the last several months. His family physician was astute enough to run some tests that found something abnormal in his abdomen. Yet he had no answers and referred him to me.

"Doc, I'm in your hands." His handshake was strong. It is always humbling when a patient walks into my office, vulnerable and searching for life-altering answers from someone he or she has never met.

Mr. Flint had retired a few months earlier at age sixty-eight from a job he had held for thirty years as a foreman at a gas company. No stranger to hard work, he was very much looking forward to his "golden years." He'd had his first job as a paperboy at age nine. He'd worked throughout his teens, giving his parents every cent he made to help keep the utilities on for him and his five siblings. He completed high school but could not afford college. Instead, he enlisted in the navy and served his country honorably. Upon returning home, he took a job with the gas company and married his high school sweetheart, Elaine. Together, they raised four loving, successful sons. They had recently celebrated their forty-fifth wedding anniversary. Mr. Flint had done all the right things in life. He was a self-made man. He was now looking forward to traveling with his wife, enjoying the Florida sun, and playing a lot of golf. That day, he and his wife were in my office looking for some answers.

"Mr. and Mrs. Flint, it's a pleasure to meet you. Tell me, sir, what has been going on the last several months?" His wife would not let go of his hand. As he spoke, I listened while reviewing the blood and x-ray test results in his chart.

"Doc, I can't put my finger on it. Just haven't been feeling well lately. I feel tired all the time. I have no appetite, lost a few pounds. My wife is getting upset because she thinks I don't like her cooking anymore." He looked at her and she smiled nervously, squeezing his hand tighter. "I have no pain." They both were worried.

"Mr. Flint, how much weight have you lost?" My eyes were still analyzing the various reports.

"About twenty pounds." I did not respond. Unexplained weight loss always raises a red flag in someone who had previously been healthy. It is a sign of something more ominous lurking beneath the surface. Prior to these symptoms, Mr. Flint had been in good health, getting regular checkups. He had a clean colonoscopy two years ago. He had quit smoking thirty years ago, was not overweight, and tried to exercise regularly. His diet wasn't always the greatest, but over the last several years he had tried to eat more of the "right" foods.

"Okay, sir, please take off your clothes and get up on this table." My physical examination of Mr. Flint revealed no clue as to what was going on with him. No pain, no physical findings, no nothing.

"Doc, what do you think is going on?" I could sense the fear in the question. I wasn't ready to be blunt with him yet. I had some ideas but needed a few minutes to prepare him and his wife for my answer.

"Mr. Flint, I have reviewed your test results. Most are within normal limits. The one abnormal report is the C.T. scan of your abdomen and pelvis. There is the *suggestion* of a mass the size of a nickel close to the midportion of your small intestine. Everything else inside your abdomen looks fine." I tried to balance the bad news with some good news. "I don't know what the mass is or how it got there." I showed him the official report. There was a long silence.

"Doc, is it cancer?" Finally, it was out in the open. He could not hold the fear in any longer. It had been the only thing on his mind since the minute he walked into my office. I paused and was glad he had said it first. "Doc, is it cancer?" I wasn't ready to confirm his deepest fear. I wanted to leave the door open for some hope.

"Mr. Flint, I don't know. It may be a tumor, it may be some inflammation, or it may be nothing at all. There are no more tests to do at this point."

"Whatever it is, can you remove it?" He didn't waste any time.

"Mr. Flint, it is possible." I could sense the frustration in their eyes, the frustration of my ambiguous answers. I could sense the fear of not knowing, the fear of his family history of cancer knocking at his door. Mr. Flint wanted desperately to get into his retirement in good health. "I won't know until I get in there, sir. You will need an operation to find out what this is and if it is removable." For the next twenty minutes, I painstakingly went over the exploratory operation I planned to carry out and the risks involved. I needed to explore the inside of his abdominal cavity to get answers. In Mr. Flint's case, the best approach would be to make a small incision and look in with a laparoscope. He had a virgin abdomen (no previous surgeries, hence no scar tissue) and was an ideal candidate. I wanted to avoid the pain and long recovery of a big incision. I wanted to avoid the trauma of a large operation in anticipation of what I might find. Based on his symptoms, I sensed I was going to find something very ominous in his abdomen. My primary goal was to get an answer without setting him back, without causing him any additional harm. I also sensed that my role as a surgeon would be minimal in his future treatment.

Mr. Flint had undergone all the right tests, but none had revealed the truth. I went over the laundry list of possibilities of what I might have to do, depending on what I found at the time of surgery.

"Mr. Flint, I might have to remove some of your small or large intestine. There is even a small chance of a colostomy." He and his wife didn't move. They just listened. I wasn't sure how much, if any, was sinking in. Most of the time, the word *cancer*, when it's first spoken, paralyzes patients. Its initial impact is so powerful, most words that follow don't register. For twenty minutes they listened as I outlined a plan. Both were now held hostage to the word *cancer* and would not be set free until my scalpel gave them an answer.

After I finished my explanation, I could see Mr. Flint's demeanor change. The can-do mantra he lived by was surfacing. He wasn't going to allow the unknown or the word *cancer* to hold him hostage. "Doc"—he looked me in the eye—"my life is in your hands. Let's do it."

Two weeks later, Mr. Flint and I had a date in the operating room. My plan was to make a half-inch incision and place a long, thin laparoscope inside his abdomen and look around. This was the best approach for him. Once inside, I would be able to determine whether this mass near his small intestine was removable.

"Okay, Nurse, this is the moment of truth. Let's see what we are dealing with." Mr. Flint was asleep, paralyzed, and breathing by respirator on the operating room table. His abdomen was sterilely prepped with an antiseptic and neatly draped off with towels. I made my incision and began to insert the laparoscopic camera inside his abdomen.

"We're in. Let's insufflate with gas and see what we have." All eyes were glued to the large television monitor connected to the laparoscope. The gas insufflation was necessary to create a space for me to work inside his abdominal cavity. I left the camera inside as the space was enlarging. As the space got bigger, more of Mr. Flint's organs came into focus. I was afraid to look.

"Doctor, what is that?" All of Mr. Flint's intra-abdominal organs were now exposed. The scrub nurse pointed to small dots scattered on the screen. I looked up slowly and came face-to-face with what I had feared the most.

"Son of a bitch." My heart sank right down to the floor as my eyes remained riveted to the television screen. I wanted to look away, but the surgeon in me was mesmerized. My biggest fears were staring me in the face. The answer to Mr. Flint's symptoms, his *not feeling right*, was clear and in high definition. There was no escaping it. He had metastatic cancer. I was eyeball to eyeball with death, Mr. Flint's death. His mortality was three feet in front of me, dots on a television screen. In several weeks, those dots would turn into more doctors' appointments, toxic chemotherapy, vomiting, pain, more weight loss, despair, and death.

"The poor bastard." I had to step back from the operating room table. "So much for retirement. How am I going to explain this to his family?" The white dots on the screen were not dots at all. They were living cancerous tissue called tumor implants.

As I quickly scanned the remainder of his abdominal cavity, more dots came into focus. They smothered the surface of every organ, choking the life out of each one. It was as if a cancer bomb had exploded inside Mr. Flint's abdomen, spraying tumor shrapnel in all directions. In these situations, the origin of the cancer is often never found. Whenever it started to grow, something caused tumor cells to break off and implant everywhere. By the time the diagnosis is made, life expectancy is short. None of the tests performed before surgery were accurate in revealing the horror in Mr. Flint's abdomen.

"Not much we can do here. It has already spread." I couldn't even find the mass suggested on the C.T. scan among the crowd of tumors pressing on his intestines. Sometimes, C.T. scans don't even come close to telling the whole story, especially with the diagnosis of cancer. X-rays can only pick up so much. These tumor implants are so small, they often never show up. "I just need to get enough tissue to confirm the diagnosis and get out. As a surgeon, I am no use to him now." As a human being, I might be able to help later.

I liked Mr. Flint. He reminded me of my father, who had passed away of cancer around the same age. Removing enough tissue to obtain a diagnosis was easy on Mr. Flint. It did not take long and he would be able to return home today. The most difficult part of my job was just around the corner, in the surgical waiting room.

As I approached the waiting room, I rehearsed the words in my head, what I was going to say to the Flint family. I hated this part of the job, hated to be the messenger of despair. I hated to deliver the worst possible answer to the question. I also hated it for another reason, a selfish reason. Give me a simple hernia to repair or an inflamed appendix to remove any day of the week. These problems are easy to fix and the outcome is easy to explain to patients and their families. "Yes, your husband is doing fine. The surgery went well. His appendix is gone and he will live happily ever after." Common problem, simple solution, good outcome, and a very satisfied patient.

I wanted to be realistic about what I had found and their father's prognosis. Yet I wanted to offer some hope, some optimism that other treatments might be effective in prolonging his life. As soon as the family saw me coming, they all stood up and nestled around their mother.

"Mrs. Flint, your husband is fine." I was trying hard to disguise the disgust in my voice. I was disgusted at the diagnosis, disgusted at the cancer's advanced stage, and disgusted at my inability to do a damn thing about it. I was also disgusted with whatever greater being forced good people like the Flints to experience the long, painful road ahead. It was just not fair. "He is in the recovery room. You will be able to see him shortly."

"Dr. Ruggieri, what did you find?"

I swallowed hard. "Mrs. Flint, your husband has cancer." There was no way of finessing this. I had to get it out there. Mrs. Flint had to sit down. She could not speak.

"Dr. Ruggieri, did you get it all?" The oldest son was now engaged.

"No, I am sorry. The disease was too far advanced. I did perform a biopsy to confirm the diagnosis. There was nothing else surgically I could do."

"Why, why couldn't you remove it?" I did not want to get into a lengthy explanation as to why it was impossible to remove. Now was not the time.

"Why wasn't this picked up sooner? My dad has always been healthy. He always went for his regular checkups. Why didn't any tests pick this up sooner?" I could see the frustration building in his face, realizing the seriousness of his father's prognosis. I could sense that he thought the medical system had failed his father, that I had failed his father by not providing answers early enough. In some ways the medical system did fail his father by not providing a method of detection early enough to impact his prognosis. Despite all the sophisticated, expensive technology at our disposal, cancer can be a very elusive demon.

"Doctor, where do we go from here?"

Mr. Flint recovered from his operation uneventfully. He began treatments with chemotherapy and radiation, attacking his cancer with the steely determination he attacked life. Despite all the mental and physical pain, his optimistic outlook never wavered. Mr. Flint succumbed to his disease one year after I gave him the answer he was searching for.

Chapter 7

———— /// ————

This Won't Hurt a Bit

"Damn, Doc, that hurts." Joe flinched as I pushed the needle into his neck, squirming toward the edge of the table. "I thought you said you were going to numb it first. What are you trying to do, kill me?"

"I'm sorry, Joe. I put some lidocaine in there, but I guess it didn't take." I reached for more, refilling the syringe. "Please, just be still for a few more minutes." I was in a hurry to get the biopsy over with. I had to be in the operating room in an hour and had an office full of patients to see later in the afternoon. I did not have the time to massage him through this.

"I hate needles." Joe winced as I injected more lidocaine underneath an area of skin along the front of his neck. "How would you like it if I stuck a needle in your neck, Doc? Hurry up, will you?" The wincing eased up. He was beginning to relax.

Paul A. Ruggieri, M.D.

"I wouldn't like it, Joe, but this has to be done. I'm going as fast as I can." I knew it wasn't easy lying flat, head arched back, trying not to take deep breaths while I stuck a four-inch needle into his neck.

"Doc, are you sure I need this biopsy?" He sounded skeptical. "I have no pain. I didn't even know I had this *growth* in my thyroid gland." He exaggerated his pronunciation of the word *growth* as if to say he wasn't convinced it existed. His eyes were squeezed shut. He went on, "I go to my family doctor for one thing and after a million tests and appointments, he finds something else. But he still can't explain my stupid cough."

"Joe, please stop talking so I can finish this. I don't want to stick this thing in your trachea. It's almost over." He was still squirming. No matter how much anesthetic I injected, he complained every time the needle went in. I passed my needle quickly through the mass multiple times, ignoring his comments with each stroke. There was nothing else I could do.

"Doc, is it over?"

"Yes, it is for now."

It really wasn't over. Joe's pain was only beginning.

Joe had shown up in my office two weeks earlier for an evaluation of something abnormal found on an x-ray. A chronic cough for several months with no apparent cause had prompted him to see his family doctor, who eventually put Joe through a battery of blood tests and x-rays. Each visit to his doctor had ended with Joe leaving with a slip of paper in his hand, yet another test order. On some appointments, Joe's doctor saw him; on other occasions his physician's assistant did. But no matter who saw him, on each visit a new test was ordered. Despite the blood work and x-rays, nothing was found that would explain his cough. That was the good news. The bad news was that one of the tests discovered a growth in his thyroid gland.

"Hello, Joe. I am Dr. Ruggieri, a surgeon." I shook his hand as I introduced myself. "Do you know why you are in my office?" I always start with this question to find out where to begin with patients.

"Doc, to be honest with you, no, I have no idea." He paused. "It has to do with needing a biopsy of a growth in my neck. It was something my doctor found. He ordered so many tests, he was bound to find something!"

Many of my patients have no idea why they are in my office. They are herded in like sheep, following orders from a family doctor on blind faith. "I finally got a call from my doctor's office telling me they were setting up an appointment with a surgeon," Joe continued. "I asked, 'A surgeon? Why a surgeon?' Of course, no one in his office would tell me."

I just listened. I knew why Joe was in my office, knew why his family doctor had sent him to me.

"First of all, Doc, it took them weeks to call me back with my test results. When the woman did, she wouldn't even tell me what they were. She said, 'Your doctor has to tell you.'" The frustration was building in his voice. "I asked to speak to my doctor, but he was busy. The woman said he would call me back later in the day. Do you think he called me back?"

I proceeded to ask Joe some questions about his health, focusing on symptoms related to his neck and thyroid gland. I also asked about a family history of any cancer. Once the questioning was done, I asked him to take off his shirt so I could examine him. While I was examining Joe, my mind was thinking ahead. I wasn't sure how much I wanted to reveal regarding my true thoughts on his problem. I needed more proof to support my suspicions.

The physical examination is by far the oldest and most traditional test any doctor can perform on a patient. It is one of the few painless tests I perform. You are not forced to drink liquid chalk, tolerate tubing snaked up your rectum, or lie still for one hour cramped in a claustrophobic cylinder with barely enough room to breathe. An examination performed by a pair of competent physician hands, a working stethoscope, and an astute mind can reveal important clues about the severity of any patient's illness. When I was a medical student, my professors relished the hours spent sharing their pearls of experience on the secrets of performing a thorough physical examination. To them, this rite of passage represented the continuation of the oldest technique in medicine. Surprisingly effective, the physical exam can still be the best window to a patient's illness. My mentors trained in a different era, when C.T., M.R.I., and P.E.T. were just letters in the alphabet. They thought differently (and dressed differently, too) than the new doctors coming out of training today. They had to rely on their ears, hands, and minds when deciding to operate on a patient. To them, ordering blood or x-ray tests was a sign of weakness.

When I became a medical student, one of my most eagerly anticipated moments was purchasing my own black doctor's bag.

I needed it for my physical diagnosis class, in which I learned the art of the physical examination. I salivated at any opportunity to show off my doctor's bag and the exam instruments inside it to anyone who might be impressed by them. The bag (along with the short white coat) validated who I was. *I am an all-knowing doctor. Here is my doctor's bag. Here is my stethoscope. I now have the legal authority to listen to your heart, and look into your eyes and ears. I also have the legal authority to place my hands on your neck, chest, and abdomen without getting arrested. I have this authority, despite not really knowing what I am listening to, looking at, or feeling.*

As a medical student, the black doctor's bag gave me self-confidence. It represented knowledge, prestige, and the $25,000 a year I was spending on tuition. It was just plain cool. Once my internship started, the black doctor's bag quickly became a second-class citizen. During surgical training, I had no time to sleep, never mind carry around a black bag filled with instruments that I had no time to use. It often got misplaced. I once left it on the roof of my car, driving home one night after being up for a day and a half on call. It was waiting for me in the same spot the next morning, perched on the roof of my car. When I became a resident surgeon, the bag ended up being not cool. I had graduated from it. I was now a surgeon. All I needed was a scalpel blade.

I still have my doctor's bag today. It is retired, tucked away in my attic and filled with corks from wine bottles of dates past. The original stethoscope and exam instruments are long gone—bargains at one of my mom's yard sales.

In today's world of specialists, the art of a thorough physical examination has become a casualty of technology. It has also become a casualty of the five-minute office visit. Sadly, its role in diagnosing illness has been supplanted by computerized imaging machines, machines that press, prod, squish, and contort every part of your body. These imaging machines will speak to you; tell you when to breathe, let out gas, swallow, and move. Some even perform surgery. It is bad enough that technology has replaced some of my ability to diagnose disease. Now, it may even replace me in the operating room.

As a surgeon, I do not spend an inordinate amount of time performing a thorough physical examination. It is not necessary for what I do. I am not interested in looking into your ears or listening to your lungs. I am interested in what I can remove. By the time you show up in my office, you have already had multiple tests. My examination is targeted toward the problem that has led you to me. If you have a bad gallbladder, my hands will be on your upper abdomen. If it's a hernia, my fingers will be in your groin. If you have a bowel problem, one of my fingers will be politely introduced to your rectum. If it's a thyroid mass, my hands will be around your neck. In Joe, I could feel a mass on the right side of his thyroid gland. It was firm and fixed, both worrisome signs for cancer. His lymph nodes were not enlarged. This was a good sign.

"Joe, one of the x-ray tests, a C.T. scan, found a growth on your thyroid gland. The ultrasound performed after that confirmed the growth to be real." Ultrasound is the best test to evaluate thyroid nodules.

"What the hell is a thyroid gland?" I pointed to the front of his neck and drew a picture to explain things.

"Joe, your thyroid gland is shaped like a butterfly. It has two sides, called lobes. The gland produces a hormone that controls just about everything in your body. The C.T. scan of your chest discovered this growth accidentally." I showed him the report. "It's just under two inches wide and needs to be biopsied." I always show my patients their reports, especially those who are going to require surgery. Most have never seen them before.

He paused, running his hand through his hair. "I was sent for tests looking for the cause of my cough and come away with a thyroid mass?" His tone became more serious.

"What do you think it is?"

"Joe, I don't know," I said.

"What do you mean you don't know? You see this stuff all the time. Why did I have all those tests? Didn't any of them tell you what it is?" I could hear the anger and fear in his voice. He was already mad at his family doctor for putting him through scores of tests and extra co-pays, with nothing to show for it. Now, he was getting pissed off at me.

"Joe, I will have to biopsy this—" He quickly cut me off.

"Doc, is it cancer? Is this thing in my neck cancer?" I wished I had an answer for him. I wished the answer were *no*.

"Joe, I don't know yet. This is why I have to do a needle biopsy. I have to get some cells from the nodule to determine if cancer is present." I had my suspicions based on the way it felt. I wasn't ready to share them with Joe until I had physical proof.

"Doc, cancer is everywhere. It was something I thought other people get, not me." He was nervous.

"Thyroid nodules are very common in the population. Autopsy studies have shown that almost half of the population have thyroid nodules when they die. Over ninety percent are benign. The odds are very good this is not cancer, but I need to prove it." I could see his relief.

"What does the biopsy involve?" He was softening his stance.

"I will guide a thin needle into the nodule, move it around, and suck up some thyroid cells. I will have to go in with the needle four times. I promise I will numb the area as best I can." I tried to make it sound routine and virtually painless. "It won't be bad."

"That's easy for you to say." The frustration was bubbling to the surface again. "You guys are all alike. You say it isn't going to hurt, but it always does. Why do you doctors always leave out the painful part? You're in a hurry to operate." He paused. "You know, Doc, my neighbor went into the hospital for a biopsy and never came out. They hit something bad, something that bled. He never recovered." Joe was getting tired; the conversation was wearing him down.

He was right. At times, I am as guilty as the next surgeon of minimizing a patient's expectation of pain in advance of a procedure or operation. It's something I do automatically, involuntarily. Maybe I have had to become insensitive to the pain I inflict. Maybe I think I am so good at performing biopsies, it would be impossible for any patient to experience pain. I know, subconsciously, I might frighten patients away if I get into the details of the potential pain in their future. And I've learned that some patients don't want to hear the fine details and some want to know everything.

"Listen, Doc, you guys have been trying to kill me for years. I have had four operations in the last fifteen years and am still kicking." His sense of humor was coming back. He was finally ready to surrender to me. "Do what you have to do."

"Good. I promise I will not be the one to kill you."

Joe's biopsy went well. He was surprised how little pain he felt by the time it was over. The anxiety leading up to the biopsy was worse than the actual procedure. It took five days for Joe's biopsy results to find their way to my desk. The results were ready earlier but I was too busy to call him. Most results from blood tests I order for patients are back within two days, not two weeks. As for x-rays, an official report is often ready within twenty-four hours. All physicians, including me, have the ability to inform patients of test results within days if they try hard enough. The potential is there. There are times when I cannot track down a result, and I pick up the phone. There have been times when I have completely forgotten about the test results, reminded only by staff or a phone call from the patient. No news is not necessarily good news. Despite lapses, I do try to inform patients of a test result as soon as I have it, especially when there is a question of cancer.

Biopsy results, on the other hand, can take longer to come back. It takes longer for a pathologist to make a final diagnosis on a piece of tissue than for a radiologist to read a simple x-ray. It is difficult to speed up this process. There is more involved in analyzing human tissue. There are times when biopsy results take a week or even longer, especially when a second opinion is involved.

I was in my office reviewing patient reports when Joe called for the second time, looking for his biopsy results. I glanced at his report. *Shit. He is not going to be happy with this.*

"Dr. Ruggieri," my secretary shouted, "Joe Jura is on the phone. He wants his biopsy results."

"Tell him I am with a patient, Annie. I will call him back." I wasn't ready to speak to him yet. I had not figured out what I was going to tell him over the phone. Plus, I was hungry and had to go to the bathroom. I feel bad (briefly anyway) when I ask a member of my staff to tell a patient something other than the truth. This wasn't the first time and would not be the last. There are times when I am not yet ready to talk to a patient or return a phone call, especially if the news is bad. There are times when I don't feel like talking. In Joe's case, technically, I was *with a patient* since I was reviewing someone else's test results. I just wasn't *physically* with that patient when he called. I went to the bathroom, grabbed a quick bite from the lunchroom, and dialed Joe's number.

"Joe, Dr. Ruggieri calling back." I wasn't looking forward to his reaction.

"Doc, thanks for calling." Silence.

"Joe, your biopsy results are in. Your thyroid nodule is a tumor but I cannot tell from the biopsies whether it is benign or cancerous. The cells under the microscope are suspicious but not conclusive for cancer. The bottom line is you will need surgery to remove the growth, along with part of your thyroid gland. It's the only way to determine if this thing is cancerous."

"What do you mean, you don't know if this is cancer?" I remained silent. At this point, he wasn't in any state to hear anything I had to say. "I thought that was the purpose of sticking those needles in my neck, so you could get an answer. Now you are telling me you don't know?" He clearly was at the end of his rope. I didn't blame him. After months of tests, he still didn't have answers.

"Joe, this is what I want you to do." I wanted to end this conversation in a hurry. "Come to my office tomorrow and I will talk to you more about the surgery, face-to-face."

"Do I have a choice?" Joe was mentally exhausted.

"No." I was mentally exhausted, too.

"I'll be there." The entire ordeal—the tests, the uncertainty, the needles, and now the worrying about cancer—had taken a toll. And it wasn't over. I felt bad for Joe, felt bad for the mental pain he was experiencing. I felt bad because I would now have to add more pain, physical pain by putting him through an operation. I felt bad, for a few minutes, until my phone rang again.

"Dr. Ruggieri, Mrs. Bixby is on the line." Annie, my secretary, sounded delighted to interrupt me again. "She wants the results of her biopsy."

Joe is not alone in his experience with the sequence of tests, doctors' office visits, biopsies, and, ultimately, surgery. I have met and treated many patients whose experiences have mirrored Joe's. All doctors order tests. I was introduced to the benefits of diagnostic tests during medical school. As a surgical resident, I was inundated with the ordering of tests and constantly challenged by tracking down the results before rounds.

Some physicians are more aggressive about ordering tests than others. I often try to restrain my impulse, because tests carry personal and financial costs, but there are times when I don't know what is going on with a patient. Times when I need help. I know tests can be uncomfortable and inconvenient, requiring time off from work. I believe every physician, to appreciate what patients go through, should experience every test we order at least once. I have not walked this walk yet. If I could choose one test to eliminate in order to avoid experiencing it myself, it would be the barium enema.

X-ray results can vary depending on who is reading the imaging films. Some radiologists, like surgeons, excel at the job. Some are better than others at reading x-rays, better at coming to conclusions. It takes time and experience for a surgeon to build trust in the judgment of a radiologist. I work with and rely on their expertise every day. Their input is often vital to me in helping to decide when to take someone to the operating room.

Test results are not 100 percent accurate. Some results are misleading, delivering false positives or false negatives. Test results can also create a false sense of security. ("See, the x-ray was negative so the problem must not be in your lungs, gallbladder, colon, or whatever organ is x-rayed.") They can be used as a crutch, an excuse for not doing some actual thinking or further pursuing the symptoms of an unexplained illness. Tests require follow-up; this takes work, especially in a busy practice.

Another reason I don't like to order tests is because I am afraid of what the radiologist may find. Medical imaging tests can reveal too much information, the so-called incidental findings. Incidental findings are described as masses, anomalies, or abnormalities in our body. Frequently, these are found by an x-ray test ordered to look for something else. Most of us are born and will die with incidental findings in our bodies, without ever knowing they existed. Many of these will remain harmless throughout our lifetime. In diagnostic medicine, incidental findings are becoming more common for two reasons: Imaging technology is more sophisticated than ever, and physicians are ordering more x-rays than ever. For surgeons, incidental findings are a pain in the ass to deal with. They can create intense anxiety in patients by giving them something else to worry about. They generate more tests (to confirm or clarify findings), often result in more pain for the patient, and generate extra (unwanted) work for the surgeon.

Radiologists reading x-rays today have a difficult job, and they inadvertently pass this difficulty on to me every time a report is generated. Their job is made difficult by the plethora of information in front of their eyes. X-ray images contain so much detail that there's tremendous opportunity for something to be missed. Technology has brought radiologists to the brink of sensory overload. It is an overload pressured by the fear of missing something, the fear of missing a cancer.

The treatment of cancer is big business in this country, nearly doubling in the last twenty years. It is big business because the diagnosis, treatment, and follow-up of a cancer generates a lot of income for hospitals and doctors. Much of this income comes from blood and x-ray tests. I recently ran into an oncologist colleague of mine who was lamenting what she has to put many of her patients through.

"Many of my patients complain of all the tests I have to put them through after their cancer has been treated. Even after they have been cured." She continued. "Once you have a patient with a known diagnosis of cancer and an abnormal finding on any x-ray, every radiology report comes back with the words,

Cannot rule out metastatic cancer, consider additional testing. It doesn't matter if they have been cured or not. It doesn't matter whether it has been five or ten years since their initial diagnosis. It doesn't matter whether, based on my judgment, I think the findings are real or not. Once those words are printed, the genie is out of the bottle. I am forced to order more tests and put my patients through more inconveniences.

"The reality of it is you have no choice. You have no cushion to rely on your judgment, not today. Maybe twenty or thirty years ago, yes, when all these tests didn't exist. Today you're damned if you do and damned if you don't.

"Official, printed reports of abnormal results also create incredible anxiety in cancer patients and their families, regardless of what I say to them." I could see her frustration. "I have never seen it this bad before. It's a never-ending cycle."

"I agree. How do you think I feel when I have to put someone through an operation just to prove that something printed on an x-ray report was not true?"

In today's practice climate of fear of missing something or getting sued, radiologists are under incredible pressure to be perfect. They are pressured to cover their asses from lawsuits with every image they read. They are pressured to comment in the official record on radiographic *abnormalities* that may have no clinical significance. In many situations, they are pressured to comment on the *possibility* of a mass showing up and the *possibility* of it being cancer. Today's imaging report findings are full of words like *possibility*, *probability*, and *rule out*, words that drive me crazy. A printed report with findings described with these words has a live patient attached, sitting in my office want-ing answers. Radiologists can do only so much with a report. They do not operate. They cannot anatomically prove what they radiographically report. I do not blame them for the way they do their job. I despise the legal black cloud they live under while they do their job. Once a radiologist's job is done, someone has to determine if the findings are real. Someone has to use another technology to find the truth, to prove that the *abnormality* doc-umented is not cancer. That someone is often me. That technol-ogy is often a scalpel blade.

Mammograms are the poster children for the painful cycle of sophisticated imaging technology, the fear of missing something, the fear of getting sued, and reports full of words covering all pos-sibilities. It is a known medical fact that too many breast biopsies are performed in this country because too many *abnormalities* are being reported on mammograms. Are these abnormalities real? In the eyes of a radiologist they are. Are most of them benign? Yes. Are all described by terms that originate out of the fear of missing an early cancer, out of fear of being sued? Yes. Who gets to deter-mine the real answer? I do. How? With a biopsy or surgery.

Most breast biopsies performed on women will reveal benign results and may not be needed. Many, I believe, are performed out of the fear of missing an early cancer and the medical and legal consequences. It is a fear that starts with the family doctor. A fear that continues its infection to the radiologist and then finally spreads to my office. In the past, I often performed biop-sies because my hand was forced by a radiologist's report stating the possibility of an abnormality, the possibility of cancer. Once the words *Rule out cancer* or *Biopsy recommended* are printed in an official mammogram report, I have two choices. The first is to use my own clinical judgment based on the merits of what was found, and observe in close follow-up with a repeat mammogram. This choice has its risks to the patient and to me. The second choice is easy. It gets me an answer in days, eliminates the risk of delay, removes fear, and eliminates lawyers from the process. That choice is a surgical biopsy, accompanied by its risk of infection, scarring, pain, lost work days, and financial hardship to the patient and the healthcare system. In reality there is only one choice for many surgeons—a surgical biopsy. It does not matter how convinced I may be, based on my clinical judgment, of the benign nature of the abnormality. Once the word *cancer* is in print on a report, fear inevitably infects my decision-making process no matter how hard I try to fight it off. Fear disrupts my thinking and causes me to cast doubt on my own judgment. A delay in the diagnosis of breast cancer continues to be one of the most common causes of medical lawsuits in the United States today. When an abnormal mammography report is in my hands and a live patient is sitting across my desk, what choice do I have?

There are many reasons I order tests for a patient. The main reason is to maximize the chance of obtaining a good surgical outcome. Before I take someone to the operating room, I want to be in a position to ensure the best outcome possible. Imaging tests can often help by confirming my suspected clinical diagnosis, or they can lead me down a different diagnostic path. Good outcomes make me very happy. They make me sleep well at night. Good outcomes result in healthier, satisfied patients.

Healthier, satisfied patients result in satisfied referring physicians. Satisfied referring physicians result in more business, and more business makes me even happier.

There are other reasons I order tests. I will order additional tests to strengthen my argument for *not* operating on a patient. Not everyone who walks into my office needs an operation. (Other surgeons may beg to differ.) In fact, many leave my office without ever going under the knife. Then there are patients whose illnesses are black-and-white, easily treated with an operation. If, for instance, the problem is colon cancer, the solution is to remove a segment of colon, no questions asked. If it is a thyroid cancer, the thyroid needs to go. The cancers I diagnose often have a straightforward solution: an operation.

There are other illnesses that, in my judgment, fall into a gray zone once all the testing is done. In these instances, an operation may or may not help. In this group, test results can be confusing, with unexpected, conflicting findings. Here, I have to use my judgment to decide whether the pain of an operation is the price to pay to get well. Then there are patients who show up in my office with a big *STOP—Do Not Enter!* sign on their body. Other patients are high medical risks, patients whose test results do not fit their symptoms, and patients whose illnesses are beyond my surgical abilities.

Some patients are referred to me because their primary care doctor does not know what to do with them. Many hope that an operation will fix what no one else has been able to figure out. *I have made an appointment to see a surgeon.* That sounds very definitive. A surgeon can always get to the bottom of things. *If*

I am seeing a surgeon, I must need an operation. But what if I don't know what to do with you? I have had patients whose symptoms I cannot explain. If I cannot explain them—with all the testing available to me—an operation is often not the answer. In my mind, most of these patients do not need surgery, despite what other opinions may state. Tests may not get me answers to a patient's symptoms, but negative results give me the courage to say, *I do not want to operate on you.* In today's world of competitive second opinions, another surgeon with yet another test result may see things differently.

I believe there are many subconscious reasons physicians order tests. Ordering tests makes doctors feel good about themselves. *Yes, I am trying to get to the bottom of your symptoms, despite not knowing what the hell is going on.* There can be a financial motivation as well. Tests generate income for physician-owned facilities and for hospitals that own physician practices. There is no denying that tests, lab work, x-rays, and other diagnostic procedures are big business. Ordering tests to investigate an illness also buys me time to allow nature to take its course.

Despite all this, I believe the overwhelming reason physicians order tests can be summed up in two words: *defensive medicine.* In a recent study, Harvard University researchers estimated that the nation's medical liability system accounted for $55.6 billion (that's 2.4 percent of all healthcare dollars spent in 2008). The medical liability system includes the cost of malpractice insurance, administrative fees, legal fees to defend lawsuits, payment settlements, and, most of all (close to $46 billion), the cost of practicing defensive medicine, which the researchers define as the ordering of diagnostic tests, x-rays, and procedures in an effort to avoid being sued.

A study published in the *Journal of the American Medical Association* in 2005 surveyed physicians practicing in Pennsylvania in all specialties (including surgeons) on their clinical decisions when it comes to the practice of defensive medicine. Pennsylvania has one of the highest malpractice insurance rates for physicians in the country. The threatening legal climate there is just plain ugly for practicing physicians. Ninety-three percent reported practicing defensive medicine by ordering tests, x-rays, unnecessary consults, and procedures to cover their asses. I suspect this number is closer to 100 percent. If I were a physician in Pennsylvania, I would consider myself negligent if I did *not* practice defensive medicine, given this study. It seems to be the standard of care.

I do not need studies to confirm what I, and many community practicing physicians, already live with. Additional testing performed out of fear may offer a sense of coverage to physicians but it comes at a cost—to all. There are physical costs to patients, putting them through tests that may not be needed. There is the risk of unexpected allergic reactions to intravenous materials given during some x-ray tests. There are financial costs to patients who must take time off from work and pay the resulting rising insurance premiums. There are emotional costs to patients, who worry about what the doctor suspects (especially when the word *cancer* is mentioned) when ordering additional tests. Eventually, I will have to share some of the cost; the insurance companies limit my payments if I order more tests than other surgeons do.

Whether we admit it or not, we all practice defensive medicine.

Some of us are better at it than others. I prefer to think of it as practicing *offensive medicine*, against the threat of missing something and being punished because of it. At this point in my career, I would rather order tests on offense, fighting back against the potential threat of a lawsuit.

When I started out in practice, my naïve professional ass was exposed every time I went to the operating room. It was sticking out there and needed constant covering; I ordered tests for every patient I saw. As a young surgeon, I could not afford to blatantly misdiagnose a patient or experience a bad outcome. As I gained more experience and survived my mistakes, I learned to rely more on judgment and less on tests. I now have the confidence to squelch the urge to order more tests, stare down the insecurity of missing something, and conquer the omnipresent fear of getting sued. Maybe I am just tired of second-guessing myself, tired of covering my professional ass. A recent study from the A.M.A. revealed that six out of ten physicians over age fifty-five have been sued. Despite all my experience, studies like this continue to force me to cover my professional ass before and after I pick up a scalpel blade, as well as during the operation itself.

My patient Joe is a prime example of why too much testing can be hazardous to your health. Joe went to his family physician with one complaint and ended up in my office with an entirely different problem. Despite the battery of tests, the source of Joe's cough was never found. What was found was a nodule in his thyroid gland, an incidental nodule that had probably been present for years. Thyroid cancer can form in nodules. It is a very slow-growing cancer, rarely spreading to other parts of the body.

Most people treated for the most common type of thyroid cancer are cured of their disease.

If Joe's physician had not ordered all of those tests, desperately looking for the source of his cough, his thyroid nodule would not have been discovered. Because it *was* discovered, Joe's physician needed to send him to a surgeon for a biopsy. The ultrasound report recommended that it be done "to rule out cancer." Something had to be done. It did not matter that the chance of this nodule being cancerous was extremely small. It did not matter that most patients are cured of the common type of thyroid cancer whether the cancer is diagnosed now or a year from now. If the thyroid nodule had not been discovered, Joe would have not gone through the pain and uncertainty of a biopsy procedure. If the biopsy results had been conclusive, I would not have had to put Joe through the pain (and risk) of one final test: an operation.

The point of the story is this: Unnecessary blanket medical tests uncover findings in patients that often would never impact their lives if left undetected. On the flip side, these tests sometimes uncover something early, something hidden away that can be treated because it *was* caught early. In my practice, this is the exception. One side effect of more tests is more discomfort, and even surgery. Once something is incidentally discovered, a decision cascade is triggered when the words *Cannot rule out cancer* are printed in an official report. In Joe's case, an unexplained cough and a string of tests brought him to my office to discuss his final test: a major operation on his thyroid gland.

"Dr. Ruggieri, Joe Jura is here to discuss his surgery."

"Thanks, Annie. Just put him in an exam room." I went over

Joe's biopsy report one last time to refresh my memory before entering his room.

"Joe, good to see you." He was not happy to see me. I sat down in front of him and reviewed the report. "Joe, your biopsy cells were suggestive of a thyroid tumor but not conclusive. As I mentioned, the only way to tell if this tumor is a cancer is to remove it." Joe listened without saying a word. "What I can tell you is that eighty-five percent of the time, your type of nodule is not cancerous once it is removed." I tried to temper the bad news about an operation with some good news, his relatively low risk of cancer. He continued to listen. "Joe, do you have any questions?"

Joe looked at me and shook his head. I continued. "Joe, do you sing?"

"Sing? Only in the shower." He was kidding but looked perplexed.

"Good," I said. "Neither do I. Joe, the main complication of thyroid surgery is injury to the nerves that control your vocal cords. If I injure one or both of these nerves, your voice could be permanently hoarse and weak." Joe's eyes grew wider. "It does not happen very often, less than two percent of the time. But it is a real complication because of where your thyroid gland is."

"Doc, has it happened to you?" Joe asked.

"Yes, Joe, it has. Not often, but it has." I had to be honest with him. "If it did occur often, I would not have a thyroid surgery practice and you would be seeing another surgeon." He was surprised by my answer. I felt bad for Joe, knowing what I had to put him through. He didn't deserve this.

"Doc, two months ago, all I wanted was an answer to my

nagging cough. Now in two weeks you are going to cut my throat and remove something I never knew I had." He paused, passing his hand down the front of his neck. "In the process, I may never be able to talk again."

"Joe, I am sorry. This is the only way we will know."

"You know," he looked away, "I haven't coughed in two days."

Joe's surgery went well. I removed half of his thyroid gland and left his voice intact. In the end, the thyroid nodule was not cancerous, a conclusion most of the supportive data in the medical literature had predicted. After Joe recovered from his operation, I could finally look him in the eye and give the answer no other test had. Despite the happy ending, the answer to the incidental finding discovered on one of Joe's tests came with an emotional, physical, and financial cost. He will be reminded of this cost every time he looks in the mirror and sees the scar on his neck. The scar I gave him.

Joe's experience is not uncommon in my practice. I frequently have to make a decision to operate on a patient, a decision that comes at the end of a cascade of tests, to rule out cancer. Any major operation has its inherent risks. Surgery can lead to complications, unexpected pain, and death, even in the healthiest of patients. Heart patients are exposed to the risk of stroke or death from heart bypass surgery. Orthopedic patients are exposed to the risk of infection in their new joints or blood clots in their legs. Gynecological patients are exposed to the risk of having their ureter damaged during a hysterectomy. G.I. patients are exposed to the risk of colon perforation every time a colonoscopy is performed. My patients are exposed to the risk of bowel perforation from the instruments I use every time I commit them to a laparoscopic operation. And all of them are subjected to the risk of harm from the anesthesia. The list of risks is endless.

When I decide to take someone to the operating room, I expose that person to pain and potential risks. When that decision is made, I have to be damn sure my reasons for operating are pure and valid. I have to be sure my reason for operating is justified by sound medical fact. I have to be sure there are no other alternatives. I have to be sure my decision is not tainted by ego or money. I have to be sure because I have the potential to hurt people.

Yes, I am a surgeon. I get paid for performing surgery. If a patient is referred to me for an operation, I am expected to operate. But there are times I have to resist the peer pressure, the referral pressure, the patient pressure, and the financial pressure, and do the right thing: *not* recommend surgery. Resisting is not always an easy position to maintain. Unnecessary surgery can lead to unexpected complications, which can lead to more surgery and more pain. I can live with the pain I inflict on patients when I am convinced the reasons for operating are just. I have to. That's part of being a surgeon. I know the pain I cause patients is only temporary. What I know I cannot live with, and hope to never face, is unnecessary pain inflicted by unnecessary surgery. Every day, before I commit a patient to the risks of an operation, I look in the mirror and ask the question: Is this absolutely necessary? For close to twenty years, I have been able to live with my answer.

Chapter 8

---///---

Patients Are the Best Teachers

THE HUMAN SPIRIT

"I think I'm going to lose it." I had to step away from the operating room table for a few seconds. One gloved hand massaged my stomach; the other reached blindly for a wall. The stench was seeping through my surgical gown and gloves. "Damn." I was gasping for some fresh air. "This is bad." I started to make my way back over to Maria, the patient on the operating table. "Nurse, put more of that smelling stuff on the tip of my mask near my nose, otherwise someone else is going to have to finish this operation." The odor from Maria's open abdomen was overwhelming.

"Doctor, do you want a new gown, or another pair of gloves?" the scrub nurse asked.

"No thanks, Lori." I bumped my waist up to the edge of the operating room table. "It won't make any difference how many pairs of gloves I have on with this case." I paused for a second. "Okay, let's go. I don't want her dying on me in the operating room. More laparotomy pads." I stuck out my open right hand, grabbing a white cloth lap pad. "Ready with the bucket?" I plunged my cupped, lap-padded hand into Maria's wide open abdominal cavity, elbow deep, making a long sweep in and out.

"Doctor, that is disgusting." Lori cringed.

"I know, Lori, I know. Isn't being a surgeon glamorous? We need to get her cleaned out. Get the bucket over here." As my full hand emerged, the white lap pad was no longer visible. It looked like a large brown soft snowball. With one quick motion, I cupped another large handful of blood-stained stool out of Maria's abdomen, sweeping it into the awaiting bucket. "Lori, another lap pad please. Keep them coming. I can only breathe through my nose for so long." Maria was testing me. It was only the beginning.

Maria had come into the emergency room two hours earlier. She was in septic shock, caused, we would discover, by a life-threatening infection in her abdomen. She had been having abdominal pain for the last week but had no one to complain to. The trouble moving her bowels had been going on for several months. Finally, the pain got so bad, she called 911.

Maria was an attractive, yet troubled, forty-six-year-old woman who had been mentally challenged since childhood. Despite her early hardships in life, she lived independently and held down a steady job in the emergency room at the hospital.

Because she was *different* as a child, her teen years were difficult. Her twenties were made even harsher when the diagnosis of schizophrenia came along. In spite of all the difficulties, she always had a smile on her face and was a pleasure to be around. Now, Maria was in the operating room facing her most difficult challenge: staying alive.

"More pads please. There is a lot of shit to clean out in here." It was one of the worst-contaminated abdomens I had ever had my hands in, and I have had my hands in plenty of shit. Maria had a perforation in her distal colon. The large hole had created a wide-open window for stool to leak through, contaminating the rest of her abdominal organs. The infection was taking over her entire body. As I continued to dig through the mess with my hands, feeling for the hole, I felt something hard deep in her pelvis. "What is this?" I washed away the area with some saline solution so I could get a better look. "This feels like a cancer." I continued to wash. "It is a cancer, a large cancer invading her rectum." I took a few quick breaths through my nose. I quickly reached up to feel the surface of her liver. "Damn. She has a hard mass on the surface of her liver as well. Probably a metastasis. This sucks."

"Can it get any worse for this woman?" Lori continued to wipe off every instrument I handed her.

"Most likely, Maria will never wake up. She will probably die within forty-eight hours, no matter what I do here. If by the grace of God she does wake up, and survives, then I will be forced to give her more bad news. Stage four rectal cancer." I could hear the conversation.

Maria, you were near death's door from a severe infection in your abdomen. You fought death off bravely and after weeks in the hospital, you beat the odds. You should have never even made it off the operating room table. Unfortunately, during the operation, we discovered that you have advanced rectal cancer, with metastasis to the liver. I did manage to remove most of it, but I had to give you a permanent colostomy bag. Once you recover from the surgery, you will need to go through months of intensive treatment for the cancer. The treatment will be rough, cause you to get sick, and lose your hair. It may slow the disease down but will not eliminate it. In the end, the cancer will kill you.

"Lori, how cruel can life be?" I started to remove the segment of rectum with the cancer in it. It was not budging. "How much more can you ask a person to take?" I could see that Maria's blood pressure was dropping. "If I were her, I would not want to wake up from this nightmare."

Maria's rectal cancer had gone undetected for months. It grew insidiously inside her to a point where it completely obstructed her colon, causing stool to back up for weeks. Her colon wall ultimately succumbed to the continued pressure and blew out like an overinflated inner tube, spewing stool in all directions. Her pain must have been unbearable just before she got to the hospital—she had a perforated colon, had an obstructing rectal cancer, was in septic shock, and had an abdomen full of stool. Just one of these critical illnesses *alone* is lethal enough to kill any healthy individual. Imagine presenting with all four.

I cleaned out Maria's abdomen as best I could and removed what I could see of the cancerous segment of rectum. I managed to get her off the operating room table alive, despite her infected body's best efforts to kill her. Upon arrival in the I.C.U., she was on maximum life support. She was receiving the strongest drugs available to keep her blood pressure high enough so her brain could stay alive while her body fought off the infection.

"We're here." I announced our arrival to the awaiting nurses. "Let's get her hooked up to the ventilator, check some blood work, and see where things are." I looked over at one of the nurses hooking her tubes up to various ports on the wall above her bed and shook my head. "Does she have any family?" I asked. "I need to prepare them. This woman will be lucky to make it to the morning."

"She has a brother. He called earlier and left his phone number. Apparently they are not close."

"Thanks." I reached up to scratch my nose. "Damn, my hand stinks." The memorable sour scent of stagnant stool does not go quietly. The scent of dead, gangrenous intestine is also difficult to wash off. Both putrid scents are similar and resistant to any number of obsessive-compulsive hand-washing rituals. My hands frequently have to coddle dead, necrotic bowel in patients or scoop out stool from a contaminated abdomen to save a life. It is not one of the more glorious aspects of my job. These circumstances can easily test the limits of my senses. The reek of Maria's infection, the stench of death in the operating room, was on my hands. I knew from experience it would not be washed away easily.

Over the next several days, Maria's life hung by a thread. If I so much as sneezed near her room, her blood pressure would drop to dangerously low levels. While the infection in her abdomen was trying to kill her, the machines and drugs at my disposal were keeping her alive. Most patients this critically ill never wake up. If they do, they are usually a shell of themselves. Most are lucky to live beyond a few days after the initial insult. Maria was maxed out on life support, yet her heart kept beating. Her kidneys were shutting down, yet her heart kept beating. Her lungs were filling up with fluid, yet her heart kept beating. Her brain was in an infection-induced coma, yet her heart kept beating. The infection in her abdomen had a death grip on her, yet her heart kept beating. Despite all the antibiotics, every week I would have to reoperate on Maria to drain a newly formed pocket of pus. After every trip to the operating room, Maria's heart kept beating.

"Nurse, what is new with our patient today?" I walked into Maria's I.C.U. room. It was day thirteen of her near-death experience.

"Seizures," her nurse replied. "Today, we have seizures." Maria had started seizing early that morning. "Look, see her arm twitching like that? It was a lot worse earlier."

"Just great." I did not want to hear any more bad news on a woman who should have died twelve days ago. "Donna, I'm a general surgeon. What the hell am I going to do with seizures? Please, let's get a neurologist involved." Maria's C.T. scan showed another abscess in her abdomen, below her liver. She had been having high fevers for two days, and this was the source. "I have to take her back to the operating room to drain another abscess." Donna looked at me with a "You have to be kidding me" expression on her face.

"This woman has been in a coma for almost two weeks and is now having seizures. Do you really need to operate on her again?" We were all under a lot of stress.

"Don't blame me. I have no choice. We've come this far, and she is still alive. I have to keep trying." I dreaded going back inside Maria's abdomen. "Has her brother been in to see her?"

"No, Dr. Ruggieri. He has not been around. I don't think he can deal with all the tubes, ventilator, and sickness in this place."

Maria's third operation went as well as expected. I was able to drain a large pocket of pus beneath her liver without damaging her intestine. Recurrent intra-abdominal abscesses in Maria were to be expected, given the contamination she had at the time of her initial operation. All I could do was drain them as they formed, as long as her heart could stand the surgery. At this point, the only thing Maria had in her favor was her strong, beating heart.

Over the next several days, the seizures dissipated and Maria's fevers disappeared. From my standpoint, she was on autopilot. Medically, everything was being done to buy her body time to heal. The only thing I did not know was whether she would have a normal mind when she woke up.

By the third week, I could sense a turnaround in her physical condition. She had been improving in small increments up until this point, with normalizing blood pressure and kidney function. Now her lung function was weighing in. "Donna, what do you think about getting that breathing tube out soon?" I want the I.C.U. nurse's input on every one of my patients, especially when it comes to milestone decisions. Intensive care nurses are very in tune with their patients and often know more about them than their doctors do. Deciding to pull Maria's breathing tube was going to be one of those milestone decisions. It was a big decision because if her lungs faltered, a decision would have to be made to put the breathing tube back in immediately. If it didn't go back in, Maria would die within five minutes. Her brother was not strong enough to make that decision yet, not strong enough to decide whether to let her go or keep her alive.

"I think she'll fly, Dr. Ruggieri. She is more awake today, more with-it mentally." Donna was confident.

"I think you're right. She is definitely more alert this morning." Maria had been in a drug-induced coma for weeks. She also had been intentionally paralyzed while on the ventilator. I wanted it this way. When her mind did break through the haze, she hallucinated, grabbed at tubes, and was a danger to herself. Comatose and paralyzed: two states that make my job easier in the intensive care unit.

"Maria." I spoke directly into her ear. "Squeeze my hand." She did. "Great. We are going to get the breathing tube out today so you can breathe on your own." Her eyes looked at me. "Good," I said, standing up. "Donna, let's aim for this afternoon. Call respiratory and get this going." Despite the progress, Maria was not out of danger yet. Even if the tube was successfully removed, Maria was still a candidate for pneumonia, blood clots, a pulmonary embolus, *C. difficile* colitis, and more infections. Any one of these hospital-acquired problems could set her back.

Once Maria's breathing tube was removed, she continued to amaze us all in her ability to survive. The next week brought more improvement in every one of her organ systems. By the fourth week in the I.C.U., Maria was fully back with the living, both mentally and physically, despite the hell her colon had dragged her through. Everyone involved in her care from the beginning glowed with joy to see her eating, walking (with assistance), and making some sense. When I walked into the I.C.U. on the twenty-sixth day, I felt like the proud parent of a newborn child.

"Dr. Ruggieri, when are you going to tell her?" Donna knew it was time.

"Today. It has to be today. I cannot keep it from her any longer." I was not looking forward to this. "She has to know." I walked up to Maria's door and stopped, trying to figure out how I was going to break the news to her.

"Hi, Dr. Ruggieri." She saw me coming. "When am I going home?"

I sat down on her bed and placed my left hand on the sheets covering her thigh. I looked directly into her eyes. "Maria, I need to tell you something." She stayed very still. "When you came into the hospital almost a month ago, you were very sick. There was a hole in your colon causing an infection, and I had to operate on you emergently. You have been in the I.C.U. almost a month."

"What caused the hole, Dr. Ruggieri?"

I paused for a few seconds. "Maria, you had a blockage from a colon cancer that caused things to back up. I had to remove part of your colon and give you a colostomy." There was just no other way to say it.

"A cancer?" She let her left hand pass over the sheets covering her colostomy bag. "Did you get it all?"

"Maria, I removed what I could. You will need further treatment once you recover from all the surgery." I was not sure if any of this registered because of the blank expression on her face. Several uncomfortable minutes passed. I was out of words and wanted to leave the room. As I started toward the door, Maria spoke again.

"Dr. Ruggieri, thank you for saving my life." I stopped and was too embarrassed to turn around. I did not want Maria to see the wetness in my eyes.

"You are very welcome." Maria's heart was still beating. Part of my heart was broken.

HUMILITY

Mr. Louis Cannon had never finished high school. While he was growing up, his father, crippled with arthritis, was unable to work, so Louis had no choice but to enter the working world full-time before his eighteenth birthday. Surrounded by twelve siblings, Louis often got lost in the shuffle, never attracting much attention as a child. Despite his unsupportive childhood, Louis was an optimistic spirit; the negativity around him couldn't bring him down. He grew to be tall and athletic and loved playing basketball. He was quite good at it and enjoyed the competitive nature of sports. As a matter of fact, he attacked all aspects of life with his naïve vigor. He was not afraid of hard work, and more than once he held several jobs at a time to earn a living.

As a young man, Louis fell in love with his childhood sweetheart, Juliette. He had met his bride-to-be at a dance where she had picked him out of a lineup of other willing boys. Juliette loved to dance. It was one of her passions. The day they got engaged, he felt like the luckiest man in the world. He was excited about a life with the woman he was born to love.

Three days before they were to exchange their marriage vows, Juliette experienced a sudden paralysis of the entire right side of her body. After weeks in the hospital, Juliette was diagnosed with multiple sclerosis (M.S.).

M.S. is a debilitating terminal neurological illness that slowly kills specific motor cells, cells that control every muscle in our body. The disease can be a slow-progressing, agonizing condition, methodically taking away every bodily function, muscle by muscle, over the years. When Juliette was diagnosed, very little treatment existed. Most patients were sent home by their doctors to die. As M.S. progresses, you become a prisoner locked in your own short-circuited body, eventually unable to move, totally dependent on others for your most basic needs.

I was introduced to Mr. Cannon when he was seventy-two years old. He walked into my office, in need of an operation. He had been referred to me by his primary care physician and on the advice of his niece, who worked in my office. Mr. Cannon was trim, tall, and handsome. He looked like he could still lace up the sneakers and hit the hardwoods with the over-fifty crowd. He had been having some vague, unexplained pains in his abdomen, pains that led him to the inside of a C.T. scanner. A vague mass had been discovered deep in his abdomen. The mass was initially biopsied by the radiologist, but the results were inconclusive. I needed to surgically open Louis's abdomen to get a definitive answer. In light of his past history of kidney cancer, everyone was worried about a recurrence. Everyone except Louis.

"Doc," he said with a confident voice, as he shook my hand.

"Mr. Cannon, can I have my hand back? I need it to make a living." His handshake was rock solid.

"Sorry, Doc." He smiled. "I hear you are the man with the skills, the man with the power. I really admire you for what you do. It is an honor to meet you." Little did I know at the time, the honor would be all mine.

For the next twenty minutes, I explained to him what the operation involved and how long he would be in the hospital. I talked about the mass deep inside his abdomen, in an area where he had his kidney removed years ago. It was my job to open him up, biopsy this mass, and prove that no cancer was present. It would be a big operation, keeping him in the hospital for days.

"Doc, I can't be in the hospital for five days and then laid up for several weeks after that." Louis's face was serious. "I just can't."

"Why not?" I was perplexed.

"Listen, Doc, I can't be away from my wife for that long. I just can't. I need to be there for my wife, Juliette. We have been married almost fifty years, and I can't leave her alone for that long." His eyes became watery as he stared out the window.

Since the day they were married, Louis had been Juliette's caretaker. For his entire adult life, he had dedicated himself to making the best out of whatever life brought them. He never complained, never wallowed in self-pity. He just kept moving forward, sometimes taking trips with Juliette in an old motorhome he purchased. Over the last several years, Juliette had become increasingly bedridden because of the advancing multiple sclerosis, losing all control over her bodily functions. She ended up with a colostomy for her bowel movements and another ostomy for her urine. Every day, Louis washed Juliette, fed her, emptied her ostomy bags, and dressed her bedsores. He often carried her to their couch to watch television at night. Louis was her Sir Lancelot and Juliette was his Guinevere.

"Louis, I understand. But we need to find out what this is. You will be no good to your wife if you're dead." He said nothing. "Louis, do you understand me?" I was getting upset. There was a long pause. I could see this decision was killing him.

"Okay, Doc. Give me a few days to make some arrangements with a nursing home for my wife. I'll call you when I am ready for the surgery."

"Louis, promise you will call me." I wasn't sure if he would go through with it.

"Yes, Doc. I will call you."

When Louis left my office that day, I began to comprehend the commitment this man had made to his wife many years ago, a commitment very few of us could ever approach. Nothing else mattered to Louis. His health was secondary to hers. His selfish wants and desires were secondary to hers. Juliette was his hero, his rock. He hated to be apart from her. He knew how to care for her, how to love her, and did not trust anyone else.

One week later I got a phone call from Louis. He was ready for his operation. He had made arrangements for his wife to go into a local nursing home while he was in the hospital recovering from his surgery. It killed him to do it, but he had no choice. He had to let her go for a week.

Louis had his operation, exploratory surgery to biopsy the mass in his abdomen. He did quite well and was discharged from the hospital in five days. He could not wait to take his wife home and care for her. Luckily, the biopsy results indicated the mass was benign. About three weeks later, I asked his niece (my secretary) when Louis was coming in for a follow-up appointment.

"Dianne, when is your uncle coming in to see me?" I was looking forward to seeing how he and his wife were doing.

"Oh, Dr. Ruggieri, I guess you didn't know. Juliette passed away one week after he was discharged from the hospital. She died of an infection from her bedsores." She paused. "My uncle is very depressed. The love of his life is gone. He may never come back." I was stunned. I had no idea. Louis had made it out of the hospital just in time to take his wife home to die. I felt guilty for persuading him to go through with the surgery, felt guilty for forcing him to choose between his health and his wife's.

Weeks continued to pass and there was still no sign of Louis's follow-up visit on my office schedule. I called several times but received no response. Finally, one Tuesday afternoon, I saw his name on my patient list.

"Louis, I am so glad to see you." I greeted him at the entrance door. He looked pale, beaten up. "I was so sorry to hear about your wife." He did not say a word. I motioned for him to follow me into the examination room. Louis looked a little thin, but he seemed to be recovering from his surgery well, at least physically. Mentally, he was hurting. Beyond the medical small talk, I did not know what to say to him. I was afraid to say anything. I wouldn't have begrudged him if he blamed me for taking him away from his wife. I would have probably reacted the same way given the circumstances.

"Doc"—I was so glad when his voice broke the silence—"I am grateful for what you did for me." I listened. "I have been caring for my wife over forty-nine years and could not be there for her in the end." His eyes were tearing up. So were mine. I could sense he was overwhelmed with guilt about leaving his wife alone in a nursing home.

"I am sorry, Louis, for putting you in such a difficult position." I did not know what else to say.

"It's not your fault, Doc. My wife suffered for most of her life. She was a prisoner of her own body. A prisoner in a jail cell created by this dreadful disease. We were just beginning our lives together when it hit. In the beginning, it robbed her of the blessing of having children. The doctors said it was too dangerous to risk having children, too dangerous because of the M.S." He looked down at the floor. "You know, Doc, Juliette would have made a terrific mother. She knew I wanted children and was willing to take the chance. She was willing to risk her life so I could have a son, a daughter. I could not let her do it." Louis continued to open his heart. "We did have a stretch of good years when the disease was in remission, but it didn't last. As the disease progressed, it took away everything you and I take for granted. She didn't deserve this. In the end, I was not going to let it steal her dignity. Through it all, I tried to make her life as normal as possible." He paused. "At least she is not suffering anymore." I could sense that an enormous weight had been lifted off his shoulders.

"Doc, thanks for your help. It has been an honor to meet you." He got up and started to walk out.

I was speechless. When Louis had walked into my office the first time, he told me he was impressed by the years of sacrifice it took to be a surgeon. He was impressed by the white coat, by the title *Dr.*, by the fact that I was a surgeon. As I'd gotten to know him, his life humbled me to the core. His sacrifice made me realize that the white coat, the *Dr. Surgeon* title, and all of life's perceived perks meant absolutely nothing. Louis does not own a white coat and has no *Dr.* in front of his name. Yet he is a better man than I could ever be. My sacrifices cannot begin to compare to what Louis gave up.

As he began to walk out, I was the one in awe, humbled by a man with more courage than I will ever know.

"Mr. Cannon, the honor is all mine."

THE BIZARRE

"Can you believe this x-ray?" I stared in amazement. "How can anyone do this to themselves?" The radiologist standing next to me started laughing. "This job is never boring. I couldn't make this stuff up even if I tried." We were both fixated on what our eyes were seeing. "This guy is a nutcase, and this x-ray is priceless."

"Listen." The radiologist spoke up. "I have seen some pretty bizarre things on an x-ray, and this one is right up there." He motioned to a young, attractive x-ray tech to come over and take a look, thinking it would impress her. "I don't know what you are going to do with this guy in the operating room, but good luck." The young woman came over and immediately put her hand over her mouth.

"The one thing I am not going to do is invite him over for dinner." We both laughed.

Fred was a fifty-five-year-old man who had been admitted through the emergency room the night before with abdominal pain. This was all I knew about him because I had not visited him on rounds yet. All I could remember from my phone conversation with the emergency room physician was a history of chronic abdominal pain and previous abdominal surgery. Even those memories were sketchy. He called me at two in the morning, when I was right in the middle of a deep sleep. I was barely awake enough to write the patient's name down. Barely able to read my own handwriting the next morning. After being entertained by his unique abdominal x-ray, I was very much looking forward to meeting Fred.

"Lisa," I asked the surgical nurse on the floor who was taking care of our patient, "where is Fred's chart?"

"Dr. Ruggieri," she could not hide her glee, "you must have been the lucky one on call last night to get this guy! He is waiting patiently for you to take him to surgery." She started to laugh. This was not a good sign and raised a red flag. *Stop. Do not go there.* No one in his right mind waits patiently for an operation.

"Lisa, what are you talking about? I haven't even met this man yet, never mind decided if he needs an operation."

"You will find out soon, my dear." She started walking away. "Call me if you need me." This basically meant I was on my own. She did not want any part of Fred. I sat down at the nurse's station and opened Fred's chart. I was curious to read his admitting papers and lab work for clues before introducing myself to him. To my right, there was a two-inch-thick chart with Fred's name on it, records from previous hospital admissions. Fred had been in and out of the hospital eight times in the past year for abdominal pain, with twice as many visits to the emergency room. He seemed to always be in need of pain medication. He also had had multiple abdominal operations over the last ten years, with the records disagreeing on whether it was five or fifteen. Once the number climbed above five, I began to lose interest.

In his past records were multiple notes chronicling Fred's long history of drug-seeking behavior. Despite his past denials, one of his favorite foods was narcotic pain medication. Fred loved to devour pain medication à la carte. One of his favorite pastimes was trying new doctor restaurants. It wasn't clear to me whether Fred's drug-seeking behavior was a result of the chronic pain from multiple operations or the cause of his multiple operations. Again, I did not care because all I wanted to do was to decide whether Fred needed an operation today. Patients with drug-seeking behavior, such as Fred, are extremely difficult to evaluate. I cannot get inside their head or body, nor do I want to, to figure out if their physical symptom is real. It can be difficult to get at the truth in these patients.

Throughout medical school and surgical training, I had received no formal education on how to evaluate drug-seeking behavior. Nothing in my training had prepared me for meeting Fred. Even today in private practice, there are no seminars on the latest updates in deciphering patients' potential lies about pain. I see no *Journal of the American Society of Narcotic-Seeking Behavior* on the hospital library shelves. The lessons I have learned about this group of patients have come from real experiences.

I have taken care of patients who have tried to steal prescription pads and fake my signature. I have taken care of patients who have stolen pain medicine from their own family members who legitimately needed it. I have had drug-seeking family members call in asking for more pain medicine on behalf of their "recently" operated-on mother who does not need it because her "recent" operation was more than six months ago. I have heard some of the most creative excuses about "lost" or "damaged" pain medicine prescribed after an operation.

"Dr. Ruggieri, I was leaning over and the open bottle of pills fell right in the toilet, the sink, the garbage disposal, the simmering soup, my scrambled eggs, the blender, and out the car window."

"Dr. Ruggieri, I accidentally threw up in my open bottle of pain pills."

"Dr. Ruggieri, my dog, cat, snake, cockatoo, rabbit, gecko, and piranha ate my pills."

"Dr. Ruggieri, my brother, sister, cousin, ex-husband/wife/girlfriend, mailman, milkman, and plumber stole my pills."

The creative litany goes on. I have also had patients whose

keen, precise knowledge of their own multiple drug allergies astounds me. The ones I have had the misfortune of operating on early in my career were ready with the list of lesser narcotic medications they were "allergic" to. The list is often a *Who's Who* in polypharmacy. "Dr. Ruggieri, I am allergic to this, this, this, and this narcotic. But I can take that one after my hernia operation." It amazes me how "that one" is always the strongest narcotic pill available.

Another impressive quality of drug-seeking patients is the effort many put into developing elaborate schemes to deceive me into coughing up a prescription for pain medication. Some patients wait until the weekend to accost an unsuspecting physician on call with a dramatic plea for pain medication. These patients know our weaknesses and go right for the jugular. They know that when I am on call I will not know all the patients I am forced to cover. They know I may be inclined to "not want to be bothered" by investigating the truth of a call from someone I do not know. Patients feed on my weakness to "get rid of them" by calling in a few pain pills; enough to last through the weekend so their own surgeon can deal with them on Monday. I once had a patient call me three days *before* an upcoming weekend, asking for a refill to get him "through the weekend" of anticipated pain. He knew I wasn't going to be on call and wasn't going to chance getting rejected by the surgeon who was. Although I was impressed by his ability to predict his "pain future," I was not moved to grant his request.

One of the most interesting, yet sad, lessons patients with drug-seeking behavior have taught me is the lesson of desperation. I have had patients who have done intentional harm to themselves in an effort to procure pain medicine. I have had patients pour their own urine on open sores in an effort to keep the pain medication flowing. These patients go well beyond my surgeon abilities. All I can do is try to identify them before they force me to add to their misery with an operation.

After I finished scanning Fred's old records, his clinical presentation raised a big red flag. I carried this flag with me to his room.

"Hello, my name is Dr. Ruggieri. I am a surgeon." I walked into Fred's room and introduced myself.

"It is a pleasure to meet you, Dr. Ruggieri." He did not seem to be in much pain.

"Tell me, what has been going on that brought you to the hospital?" I wasn't ready to open up the can of worms his x-ray findings conveyed. I wanted him to tell me his story, in his own words. For the next ten minutes, Fred described how he had been having intermittent abdominal pain for months. For some reason, the pain had just gotten worse that day, forcing him to come to the emergency room. He also stated that he had been operated on in the past for intestinal obstructions, the last operation carried out by one of my partners over a year ago.

"Is the pain made worse by anything? Eating?" I was trying to drag the truth out of him with open-ended questions, but he would not bite.

"No, not really, Doc. I know I have scar tissue in my abdomen from my previous operations that causes me pain. I am not sure what happened to make it worse this time. Can you operate and remove the scar tissue?" I had just about had enough of Fred. It was time to get to the truth.

"Fred, do you know you have the equivalent of a full place setting of utensils in your intestine? Do you know you have metal pins and some nails in there as well? Your x-ray revealed enough metal in your intestines to set off a metal detector fifty yards away." I paused for a response. There was none. "Fred, I would be shocked if you *didn't* have pain with all that in there."

He looked at me. "Yes, Dr. Ruggieri, I know." He did not elaborate on how it all got in there. It was obvious to both of us how the objects landed in his gut. I just did not know the why part. I did not push Fred any further as to the reasons he swallowed several pounds of silverware, pins, and nails. I did not want to go down that dead-end road before the psychiatrist had his chance. Maybe he liked the taste of metal. Maybe he was iron deficient and thought, in some twisted way, this was the best way to treat his lack of iron. Maybe he purposely swallowed objects with the goal of perforating his intestine, necessitating surgery and writing his ticket to more pain medication. It was obvious Fred had some psych issues, issues that made him think of dessert when he looked at a fork or a spoon or a nail. I wasn't there to evaluate his mind. I was asked to evaluate his abdomen. Fred's x-rays showed no evidence of a perforation.

No perforation, no operation, no pain medication. Thank you, God.

Fred was lucky this time. I was lucky this time. He did not need an operation—despite the collection of Grandma's finest silverware inside him. I did not need to operate on an abdomen with more scars than I have fingers. Cutting through the scar tissue to find the perforation would have taken hours, not to mention increased the risk for more damage to his intestine. After an operation, Fred would have been in the hospital for weeks sucking up the intravenous narcotics. It would have been virtually impossible to get him out and only a short time before he was back.

"Fred"—I wanted to be very blunt with him—"you do not need an operation from me. Your pain is from one, if not all, of the utensils you have ingested. Utensils that have become lodged inside your gastrointestinal tract. I am not going in there to fish these things out. Not going to cut away any scar tissue. An operation will cause you more harm than good." He just looked at me. "You are going to have to live with this."

"Okay, Doc. If you are not going to operate on me today, can I have something to eat?"

Chapter 9

―――――― /// ――――――

Thoughts on Death and Lawsuits

DEATH

I sat there alone at Mrs. Franklin's bedside in the intensive care unit, staring at her face. It was a face whose features were lost in the maze of blood-soaked plastic tubes suffocating every orifice. She was bleeding internally because an overwhelming infection prevented her blood from clotting. I was bleeding emotionally. I desperately wanted her to wake up. I desperately wanted her to say, *I forgive you for not operating on me sooner. I forgive you for letting my colon perforate. I forgive you for allowing my body to go into septic shock and bleed. I forgive you for the pain you have caused me and my family. I forgive you for the circumstances that have brought me to the brink of death.*

Mrs. Franklin came into the hospital with an intestinal obstruction. I was asked to evaluate her as a surgical candidate. For several days, her bowel obstruction seemed to be improving with nonsurgical treatment. I thought I was off the hook until I received the frantic call from her nurse.

"Dr. Ruggieri, Mrs. Franklin is in a lot of pain and her blood pressure is dropping." That was all I needed to hear. Instinctively, I knew what had transpired. I knew something catastrophic had occurred suddenly in her abdomen, requiring emergency surgery. I was tied up in the operating room the day before and had not had a chance to visit her. After a rushed surgery to repair a hole in her colon, I went back and reviewed her chart. There were signs, subtle signs hinting at something building the day before. Warning signs only a surgeon would be able to recognize. If I had gone by to see her the day before, I might have recognized the looming trouble sooner and acted before her body started to shut down.

This wasn't the first time I had been introduced to impending death, and it would not be the last. Death has always been an unwanted yet unavoidable component of my job. When I was a medical student, death's first arrival was emotionless, in the form of the elderly cadaver we called "Aunt Tilly." Aunt Tilly was a beautiful learning tool, nothing more. Her formaldehyde perfume and leathery skin made her not real. As medical school progressed into the clinical years, death took on a warmer presence, in the form of live patients. Despite heartbeats and stories, their deaths due to illnesses were teaching lessons, with no lasting impact or emotional jolt to me personally. As I became a surgeon in training, death evolved into something I worked at trying not to cause. Its presence during residency made some inroads with me, but its emotional impact was fleeting, even after my first encounter.

"Dr. Ruggieri, I need you to pronounce Mr. Hendricks, please." The surgical nurse grabbed me as I was leaving the floor. She had gone in to take his blood pressure and found him stiff and dead. It was two in the morning. Being the intern on call, I still had several live patients to see. The only thing I knew about Mr. Hendricks was that he had terminal liver cancer. He had been tucked away in a corner bed, waiting to die.

"Nurse, I have never pronounced anyone dead before." I needed some help.

"It's easy. Go in there, feel for a pulse, listen to his heart and lungs, and write a note. Trust me. He has been trying to die on my shift for several hours. Make sure you date and time your expiration note. I will take care of the rest." She made it sound so routine. I dreaded this moment for two reasons: First, I was not prepared to put my hands on a dead person. It wasn't on my scut list; I had blood work to track down, x-rays to see. I was focused on the living, worried about reading up on the blood supply to the stomach for tomorrow's gastric resection case. The second reason was that I was petrified of being wrong.

"Nurse, what if this guy wakes up asking for his urinal ten minutes after I pronounce him dead?" She laughed. "I'll never be able to live it down."

"Don't worry, Doctor. I will hold your hand." I looked around for a colleague.

"Okay, let's do it." I walked into Mr. Hendricks's room. "He looks dead to me." I felt for a carotid pulse. "I think I feel something."

"Are you sure?" I could tell she was getting annoyed. She was right. I was feeling my own increasing pulse. Several minutes went by.

"Can we hurry it up, please?" The nurse needed to give the man across the hall some pain medication.

"I don't think he has a pulse." My hands were sweating. I listened to his heart and lungs. "Nothing here." I listened again. "Yes, I think he is dead."

"Good. I agree. Here is the death certificate. Could you fill this out and leave it in his chart?" With that, she exited the room and left me standing there alone. I watched Mr. Hendricks an extra ten minutes, just to be sure he was dead.

Now I continued to stare at Mrs. Franklin. I was hoping her wide-open eyes would see my face. Hoping she would acknowledge my presence. The rhythmic beat of her ventilator discharging each breath jabbed at the silence. I almost grabbed her shoulders to shake her. *Wake up! Damn it, wake up! You can't die on me.* I was overwhelmed with guilt. Guilt was what brought me to her room. Guilt was what sat me down. Guilt was what had me begging for her to wake up. I felt like I had let her and her family down by not recognizing the subtle signs pointing to imminent perforation and failing to operate on her sooner. If I had, she might not be lying here, paralyzed, intubated, comatose, and fighting for her life.

Throughout my career, death has had many faces. Some, I have felt personally responsible for. When I was a young intern, death was the face of Jeff, a fifteen-year-old with burns to more than 30 percent of his body. Jeff was caught in a house fire and admitted to the burn unit. I was an intern with much to learn when Jeff arrived. Despite appearing stable, he had also suffered an inhalation injury I did not recognize. Inhalation injuries deceptively cause throat swelling. They often go unnoticed until a patient suffers a respiratory arrest. When Jeff suddenly stopped breathing, I had a difficult time getting a breathing tube in him. There was too much swelling in his trachea, too much inexperience in my hands. Jeff's brain was short of oxygen for several long minutes. I finally managed to intubate him with a breathing tube, but it came with a cost. He never woke up. Infection, blood clots, and finally death followed for Jeff. I blame myself for not anticipating his respiratory arrest, not intubating him before the crisis. His bloated face and body still haunt me today.

///

During my chief resident year, death's face belonged to Frank, a seventy-five-year-old war veteran of the Battle of the Bulge. As chief resident, I was given full responsibility for every patient I took to the operating room. As chief, I began to develop a genuine emotional connection to patients under my care. Frank had presented with weight loss, abdominal pain, and a diagnosis of stomach cancer. He was also a heavy smoker and at high risk for pneumonia. I realized I had one chance with Frank, one chance for a perfect operation and postoperative course. A setback of any kind for him would most likely be fatal, given his frail lungs. Frank's operation went flawlessly. His postoperative course did not. He developed a deep wound infection that I blame myself for. Frank had to be taken back to the operating room to have an abscess drained. This time, he never got off the ventilator. His damaged lungs did not have the reserve to carry him through the second operation. Pneumonia invaded Frank's lungs, soon opening the door to his death. The memory of Frank's body, with his incision draining pus, forever plugged into a ventilator, is still as vivid as the day I took him back to the operating room.

Now that I am a surgeon in practice, death has grown to be much more personal because there are no buffers between me and its wake. There are no textbooks, no residents or mentors to shield me from responsibility. If I operate on a patient and he or she has a complication or dies, it is my responsibility. My name is the name on the medical chart. My decision, my knife, my responsibility. As a resident in training, I always found an excuse not to face death. There were many every day. Death is very personal now, personal on many fronts. It's attached to names and faces I know.

Jane was a twenty-two-year-old woman in the last trimester of her pregnancy when she noticed a firm mass in her left breast one morning in the shower. I almost dismissed the mass as the normal breast tissue of pregnancy when I first saw her. Something inside me forced me to biopsy it. The mass turned out to be a very aggressive form of breast cancer. Jane had her pregnancy induced and underwent aggressive surgery, chemotherapy, and radiation, only to succumb in the end. Why does a young mother-to-be get an aggressive form of breast cancer and never get to see her daughter graduate high school?

Death was also George, the thirty-nine-year-old construction worker, married with two small children. George had been having some vague abdominal discomfort for months. He was ultimately diagnosed with colon cancer. He was otherwise healthy, had no risk factors, and loved his job. His cancer looked curable until I opened him up and saw the extent to which it had consumed his other organs. I removed what I could, without causing him harm. Before his abdomen was closed, I knew George would be dead within a year, regardless of the treatment he received after his operation. Before the last fascial suture was placed, emotionally I had to let him go. I had to let him go because he was only two years younger than me. I had to let him go because there was nothing else I could do. There was nothing else anyone could do. George desperately wanted to live, wanted to see his two girls grow up. He recovered from his surgery and even went back to work while receiving chemotherapy. The man had incredible stamina. Despite the treatments, George succumbed to his disease thirteen months after I entered his abdomen.

///

Death never looked so sophisticated as when I met Anna, a seventy-two-year-old woman I was asked to see. She had entered the hospital because of difficulty breathing. A large thyroid mass was discovered on her exam. Anna was a beautiful woman, even in her seventies. I could tell she must have broken some hearts as a young lady. When I came to see her, her neatly kept appearance had an aura of self-respect no hospital gown could bring down. Her speech, her mannerisms all conveyed to me a woman of sophistication.

"Mrs. Francis, it is a pleasure to meet you." I shook her hand. My eyes were glued to the mass in her neck.

"The pleasure is mine, Dr. Ruggieri. You are such a handsome doctor." She was flirting. "Please, call me Anna." I was loving it. "I hear you are the best at dealing with thyroid glands."

"Thank you." My eyes continued to sum up this very large mass along the front of her neck. It looked worrisome. I asked her a couple of questions about her symptoms, her trouble breathing, while examining her thyroid gland. "How long have you had this mass in your thyroid?" My hands were palpating it as I listened to her answers. It felt hard and fixed. Both bad signs. "Anna, has anyone informed you of your biopsy results?" Anna had had a biopsy done in radiology several days earlier. I was hoping the answer would be yes. I hated to be the bearer of bad news.

"No, Dr. Ruggieri. My other doctors have been waiting for you to see me first." A concerned look overcame her face. *This sucks. They leave it up to me to tell this woman she is going to die. I have to tell this lovely woman she has the most aggressive type of thyroid cancer known, anaplastic thyroid cancer. I have to tell her there is nothing I can do surgically for it. I have to tell her the cancer is too far advanced and is inoperable. There isn't anything anyone can do for her. I have to inform her that the disease is often resistant to any types of chemotherapy or radiation. It is a relentless cancer growing rapidly, invading the trachea and the major blood vessels in the neck. In the end, you end up with a tracheostomy, only to suffocate from the disease. It is a horrific way to die.*

"Anna, I am sorry to tell you, the biopsy was positive for thyroid cancer." She took the news with all the sophistication her outward appearance suggested. I was not surprised. "The type of thyroid cancer you have is too advanced for me to remove. There is nothing I can do to help you." This is the worst thing a patient or a family can hear from a surgeon. I was supposed to be the knight riding in on the white coat, capable of slaying the evil cancer with my knife. Most patients, once they hear the word *cancer,* ultimately focus on a cure. *Just get it out of there. You are a surgeon. Remove my cancer so I can go on living.* I wish it were that simple. Once they hear the words, "There is nothing I can do," the spirit of living, of hope, takes a big hit regardless of what comes next. To young patients and families, the words *I was unable to remove anything* are especially difficult to say and to accept. I felt impotent in the face of Anna's thyroid cancer. I felt that I had failed her without even getting the opportunity to operate.

"Dr. Ruggieri?" I was feeling sorry for her and myself. "Am I going to die?" I knew this question was coming. I did not want to answer it.

"Anna, there are some medicines that may be able to shrink the tumor. Radiation may help." She interrupted me.

"Dr. Ruggieri, am I going to die?" She knew I was trying to avoid answering her question.

"Yes, Anna." I hesitated. "You will ultimately succumb to this disease." I had to be honest with her about the final outcome. Her life, her presence demanded I be honest with her. I left Anna's room heartbroken, knowing what the future held for her.

The last time I saw Anna she was lying peacefully, wearing a beautiful dress and necklace of pearls. Her eyes were closed. I knelt beside her and said a prayer. The lipstick, mascara, and rouge on her face reminded me of an aging actress, ready to play her last part. Her hands were neatly folded around a rosary chain. She was at peace.

///

Mrs. Franklin remained in a coma for weeks, a coma I felt partly responsible for. In my mind, I knew she was never going to wake up, never going to give me the opportunity to explain myself. With each artificial breath, the reality of her physical death grew stronger. In the end, Mrs. Franklin never woke up; she died of multisystem organ failure due to infection. After learning of her death, I managed to gather the courage to attend her funeral and place myself at the mercy of her family. At the very least, I had to pay my respects to a family I believed I had let down. I also had to face my own demons and deal with the death of a patient, a death that might not have occurred if I had acted sooner.

Mrs. Franklin was not the first patient to die under my care from the consequences of a clinical decision I made. She was not the first patient I'd lost and felt personally responsible for. I mentally beat myself up over her death for some time. I could still function and continued to operate. I had to. Others relied on my skills. At the end of the day, I had to stop the emotional bleeding over the death of Mrs. Franklin. I had to allow the wound to scab over. As a surgeon, I have learned to live with the deaths I have faced. Over time, the memory of Mrs. Franklin's death found its way into the same dark room in my brain where the others are kept. This room is not crowded. I keep it locked during the day. Despite my best efforts, the door to this room does get forced open by new circumstances, reuniting me with the old faces of death I have known. When it does open, the bleeding begins again.

When I met Mrs. Franklin, I did not expect her to die. When I met Jeff the burn patient or Frank the World War II veteran, I did not expect either one to die. When I meet most of my patients, death is the furthest thing from my mind. In my early days, I never expected anyone to die. Years at my craft have made me a realist. I understand and accept the fact that some of the patients under my care will die regardless of the circumstances. I also accept the fact that some of the decisions I make (or don't make), inside or outside the operating room, may be contributing factors to a patient's death. An unexpected death, as in the case of Mrs. Franklin, is difficult to process. It is also difficult for a patient's family to accept. An unexpected surgical death leads to many questions: questions regarding the circumstances, questions regarding the surgery, and questions regarding specific aspects of care. These questions are asked not only by family members but also by me. *What if I had operated sooner? What if I held off for twenty-four hours? What if I ordered this or suspected that before things got out of control?* I am constantly questioning myself when a patient dies unexpectedly. In the end, I have to live with the decisions I make. I have to live with the fact that my decisions have the potential to save or take away life.

A former patient once asked, "Dr. Ruggieri, how do you feel after losing a patient?"

"It sucks." The first part of my answer was easy. The second part was complicated. "It also depends on the circumstances."

Katherine was a sixty-five-year-old woman who came to the emergency room in septic shock. She had experienced brain damage at birth and been a ward of the state ever since her parents gave her up. Katherine never had the chance to experience a "normal life." She was kept alive by a feeding tube and lived in a nursing home. Over the last twenty-four hours, she had been experiencing abdominal pain and was brought to the emergency room by ambulance. After I examined her, it was obvious something catastrophic was evolving inside her abdomen.

"Does this woman have any family?" I needed to prepare her family before I took her to the operating room.

"Yes, Dr. Ruggieri. She has a brother. He is on the phone." An astute nurse was smart enough to get in contact with him. I grabbed the phone from her.

"My name is Dr. Ruggieri. Are you Katherine's next of kin?" I needed to hurry.

"Yes, I am," he answered.

"Sir, your sister is very sick and needs emergency abdominal surgery. Otherwise she is going to die here in the emergency room." He listened. "There is a very good chance she may not make it out of the operating room. But her only chance is an operation."

I knew Katherine's chances of surviving were very low based on her clinical presentation. There was something dead in her abdomen. I had to get it out. An operation would probably kill her. What other choices did I have? There were no good options here. If I didn't operate, she would die. If I did take her into surgery, the stress of an operation could kill her. It was that simple. Even if I was able to get her off the table, she would probably not make it through the night. There was a long silence on the other end of the phone.

"Doc, do what you can." He did not know what to say. He lived across the country and had not seen his sister in years. Part of me was hoping he would say, "No, just let her go." Often, in patients as critically ill as Katherine, an operation is just an exercise in futility, an autopsy in the operating room. In these situations, I would rather step aside and let nature take its final course. I instinctively knew what was waiting for me inside Katherine's abdomen. I knew that even if she survived the trauma of an operation, her chances of waking up were small. Even if she did survive, what kind of quality of life would she have? I knew it would be even worse than her first sixty-five years.

Within an hour, I was inside Katherine's abdomen and came face-to-face with her death.

"Dr. Ruggieri, look at her intestine!" The operating scrub nurse knew what came next.

"Dead bowel. It's all dead." Katherine's entire small intestine was twisted in a sailor's knot, choking off its blood supply. I looked at every inch of her small intestine. "There is nothing for me to do here. This woman will be dead within an hour." After placing her blackened intestine back inside its home, I proceeded to close her abdomen with sutures. As I was closing, my mind was going over the words I would use to inform her brother. The insult to her intestine was irreversible. Her fate sealed with each twist. Katherine was already dead when she arrived in the emergency room.

After I finished closing, I picked up the phone and talked to Katherine's brother. It is painful to inform the family that a loved one will die shortly. Early in my career, I choked on the words, "There was nothing I could do." To me, these words meant I had missed something or failed to act sooner. Now, I understand and accept that some patients will die under my care. Some will die before I take them to surgery. Some will die on the operating room table. Some will die after surgery. There will be rare times that my decisions may contribute to their deaths. There will also be times that my decisions will save lives. And there will be times when I will be impotent as a surgeon. Katherine's operation was one of those times.

"Sir, I am terribly sorry. Your sister's entire small intestine was dead from being twisted. There was nothing I could remove to save her." There was silence on the other end.

"What does that mean, Dr. Ruggieri?" he asked.

"It means she will probably not make it through the night."

With Katherine, there was nothing I could do to change the course of events. It was not the first time, and it would not be the last. There will be others to follow Katherine. Some will be saved, and some will die. Some of the deaths will be expected, and some will not. I will not lose much emotional blood over the death of Katherine because her fate was sealed by whatever force caused her intestines to twist. I only have so much emotional blood to give when I step into the operating room. I am not a miracle worker. I do not pretend to be. Katherine's death will slowly fade from my consciousness—while the memory of Mrs. Franklin lying in her intensive care bed, comatose, is alive and well.

GETTING SUED

I had just returned from the operating room, having stopped a bleeding ulcer on a patient who was trying to die. As I entered my office, I could see my office manager walking slowly toward me with an envelope in her hand.

"Hi, Kathy. What a great day. I just stopped a woman from bleeding to death on the operating room table." I was drunk with satisfaction. "Days like today make it all worthwhile." I was less than a year into my practice, eager to get my name out in the community. "Who's next?" I felt invincible.

"Dr. Ruggieri, I have a certified letter with your name on it from a lawyer representing our malpractice insurance company." I felt the air leave my chest. I grabbed the envelope from Kathy. I stared at it.

"What is this? Kathy, a letter from any lawyer is never good news." I slowly opened it and started reading. *You are hereby named as one of the defendants in the lawsuit brought by Mrs. Williams for gross negligence . . .* I read on. . . . *contributing to a retained surgical sponge in her abdomen.* I couldn't read any more. "This is bullshit. I cannot believe my partner and I are getting dragged into this lawsuit." I had to sit down. "We were the ones who bailed out the son of a bitch. Don't they know that?"

"Dr. Ruggieri"—Kathy was trying to offer consolation— "lawsuits do this all the time. Lawyers will attempt to name every doctor within a mile radius of a plaintiff's chart when filing a lawsuit." I sat and listened. "They drag as many doctors as possible through the legal mud." I was less than a year into my practice, a practice not yet seasoned with cynicism or fear. I was also naïve to the long-term consequences of being named in a lawsuit. "More defendants mean more hours to bill. Lawyers know that doctors loathe being part of a lawsuit. They feed off their distaste for having to take time off to defend themselves. Lawyers know that surgeons detest being forced in front of a jury, having to justify their decisions and the care they gave." Kathy was educating me on the anatomy of a medical malpractice lawsuit. "The process is cruel. It weeds out the irrelevant physicians, while slowly tightening the noose around the neck of the main accused." As I was to learn, the process comes at a cost to all, both emotionally and financially. "Dr. Ruggieri, in the end you and the others will be exonerated by the truth." She was trying to ease the pain.

"Kathy, the actual truth is often irrelevant. The final truth ends up originating from an economic decision. The truth is this surgeon created his own problems. It took several of us to bail the bastard out. After repairing the damage he created, we left the room. We weren't even there when he closed her abdomen with the sponge inside. Two weeks later she returned with an abscess in her abdomen caused by the sponge and had to be reoperated on." I paused to catch my breath. "Personally, I don't blame her for suing. I would have done the same thing. There are some surgeons who should not be operating, despite being granted privileges. Kathy, most patients I have had complications with understand bad outcomes happen. Most are willing to accept my imperfections, despite the pain they might cause them. Most are willing to forgive and not sue if they feel I have been honest and sincere in caring for them." Kathy just nodded her head.

"Patients will sue me after a bad outcome if they feel I am ignoring their complaints. They sue if I do not spend time communicating with them. They will sue me if I come off as an arrogant S.O.B. or act like their bad outcome was someone else's fault. In the end, they will sue if the nature of the bad outcome is just too much to bear. Someone has to shoulder the blame. I invite trouble when my ego doesn't listen to my brain. I invite legal trouble when I don't know my own limitations in the operating room. I also invite legal trouble when I operate on the wrong person for the wrong reason."

"Dr. Ruggieri, this wasn't even your complication."

"I know. Why don't this woman and her lawyers recognize this? This is what I fear most about lawsuits. Any patient at any time, regardless of the quality of care given, can file a frivolous malpractice lawsuit, oblivious to the implications to those involved. All they have to do is look in the phone book or turn on the television to find a lawyer." I was getting worked up.

"Dr. Ruggieri, I think they should also reimburse you for your time lost," Kathy said.

"Good idea. If you put all malpractice lawyers on one global fee per case, instead of billing for every second they pick up the phone, they will think twice about it. Why not? This is how I get paid as a surgeon." I paused. "I realize that what happened to this woman goes beyond forgiveness. There is no excuse for leaving a sponge behind. This should not happen. But it does. It happens now and it will happen again in the future."

"Why do you think it does?" Kathy asked.

"It happens because we are too busy, we get careless, we're tired, we rely too much on others, and we're human. It happens because we cannot be perfect one hundred percent of the time in a world where perfection is required one hundred percent of the time. Do you know, despite all the new rules, operating room checklists, and 'time outs' installed in operating rooms, the number of wrong-site surgeries has increased in this country? I understand that checklists and time outs have reduced the incidence of mistakes in the operating room, but they are not perfect. Kathy, this surgeon should have manned up from the beginning, admitted his role in what transpired, and fallen on his sword. This patient was *his* responsibility. The damage was done by *his* knife. The retained sponge was left on *his* watch. It is every surgeon's responsibility to be accountable for his or her actions inside the operating room. Somebody other than a lawyer should have recognized this from the beginning. Somebody should have screened this case and gone right to the surgeon responsible. It would save the rest of us a lot of emotional grief and the system a ton of money. The system needs to change. I should have never received this letter."

As a result of two opening sentences in a legal letter, I was initiated into a secret club rarely spoken about. It is a club that brands you with a scarlet letter. A letter you spend the rest of your life trying to hide. I soon would journey through a legal process that swallows you whole, takes a few bites, and then regurgitates you. In the end, it leaves you alone to clean the emotional vomit off your white coat before getting back into the operating room.

Living through a malpractice lawsuit forever changed me. It was an early wake-up call to the reality of the practice of medicine. The day I received that certified letter was the day I lost my professional virginity. I was young; it hurt like hell, I wanted it over quickly, and I would never speak about it again. I would also be wiser when the potential for the next one undressed itself. As the lawsuit unfolded, the very foundation of my professional altruism was shaken. The entire process made me question my belief in thinking I could help and trust patients. Negligence! I could not even put my lips together to say the word.

As a defendant, I was embarrassed, shocked, pissed off, humbled, and confused. I was embarrassed because the process made me feel like I was part of some unspeakable evil. It made me feel I had purposely planned to cause harm, schemed to *be negligent* that day. I was shocked because nothing up to that point had prepared me to deal with the emotional baggage associated with being named in a lawsuit. There were no classes in medical school on how to avoid or survive a malpractice suit. When I was a surgical intern, there was no rotation in the surgical malpractice intensive care ward. I was angry at the surgeon who had dragged me into it. I was furious at the malpractice lawyers for doing what they do—making money off the honest and dishonest imperfections of physicians. I was confounded by the patient for not knowing who the good guys were. Lastly, I was annoyed with myself for being naïve enough to think, *Because my intentions are good when I enter the operating room, I am immune to getting sued.* My ego was severely bruised. Lawsuits happened to other surgeons, not me. I was also confused because I had no idea what the long-term ramifications would be on my career.

I was sure my reputation would be severely threatened, sure

that word would get out and referrals would dry up. As the suit ran its slow course, it felt like I was emotionally bleeding every time I had to devote energy to defending myself. During the long uninvolved gaps, I did my best to scab over my wounds until the next meeting or deposition. Then, the bleeding would begin again. I had never been through a deposition before and was unsure of what to expect. To this day, the only part I remember is when the lawyer for the surgeon my partner and I had bailed out accused me of causing some of the damage to the patient. It got ugly because careers were at stake.

Three years later my office manager presented me with another legal letter, this one from my lawyer. I opened it slowly. *It is ordered, adjudged, and decreed that summary judgment is granted as to the Defendants Dr. Paul A. Ruggieri . . .* The truth had finally arrived. Summary judgment meant I was dropped from the case.

"Great news, Dr. Ruggieri!"

"Yes, it is good news." I was subdued. "However, it's not over for me."

"What do you mean?" She asked.

"For the next ten years, this black mark is on my record, even though I've been dropped from the case. Every time I apply for hospital privileges or renew my medical license, I have to explain why I was sued and what the outcome was. If I move to another state and practice, I have to show documentation of what transpired and how it ended to every hospital or state licensing board. It doesn't end." With every reliving of this lawsuit, the emotional scabs get ripped off and the bleeding starts again.

What happens to surgeons who do get judgments against them? Surgeons who lose or settle a medical malpractice suit get their names permanently placed in the secret National Practitioners Data Bank, the N.P.D.B., if the judgment is more than a certain dollar amount. The N.P.D.B. is a government agency created by Congress in 1986 to improve the quality of healthcare. It collects the names of physicians who have been sanctioned by state licensing boards, engaged in unprofessional behavior, or made medical malpractice payments. The information gathered by the N.P.D.B. is not accessible by the public. Hospitals and state licensing boards granting privileges to doctors are the only entities with access to the National Practitioners Data Bank. They use the data to evaluate a doctor's competency and candidacy when granting privileges and licenses.

GETTING SUED—MORE THOUGHTS

"I cannot believe your company is unwilling to reimburse me for the cost of Mr. Thompson's physical therapy co-pays." I was pissed off. "It was a lousy two hundred fifty dollars I volunteered to pay out of my own pocket because it was the right thing to do." My voice was getting louder. "I have paid you guys close to four hundred thousand dollars over the last ten years for malpractice insurance. During that time I have worked my ass off to stay out of the courtroom by successfully taking responsibility for my complications throughout the years. Your company has had the good fortune of not having had to spend a legal dime on me for the past ten years while cashing my checks. Now you will not even reimburse me a paltry two-fifty?" I was sweating.

"No, I am sorry, Dr. Ruggieri, it is against our policy—"

"Fuck the policy." I interrupted. "You guys are all alike. You have me by the balls because of the nature of what I do. I have no choice but to pay you. Your monopoly on the region I practice in offers me no choices. You don't give a shit about the patient or doctor. I am trying to *help* this patient and avoid a lawsuit. You guys can't budge because of a stupid policy? You guys should *thank* me for saving your company thousands of dollars in legal bills. Every year my malpractice rates go up, despite my clean record. Why don't I get a refund for practicing safe surgery? Every time I get your bill I'm just glad I'm not an obstetrician paying six figures a year for malpractice insurance. I don't get a break for passing on high-risk patients or for going out of my way to correct a wrong I created. Even if I did get sued, your 'policy' dictates that I have no say if your company decides to cut its losses and settle against my wishes." I was out of breath.

"Unless Mr. Thompson contacts us directly and offers to sign a waiver stating he will not sue, I cannot help you or him." The company representative was not budging.

"There is no way I am going to ask him to call you. You're the ones that should be contacting him. No way am I going to encourage him to sign anything. The last thing I want right now is for him to even hear the word *lawsuit*. He has enough problems with the complication from my surgery."

"I am sorry, Dr. Ruggieri." The representative didn't know what else to say.

I had offered to pay Mr. Thompson's co-pays for physical therapy because I sensed he was short of cash. I felt bad about his inability to work. I felt bad about the pain in his arm.

"Hell, I am so pissed off right now I might even encourage the man to sue me. At this stage of my career, I can deal with it. At least I will get some mileage out of all the malpractice insurance money I have paid you throughout the years." I hung up the phone.

A month earlier, I had removed a suspicious lymph node from Mr. Thompson's armpit to rule out lymphoma. I thought the surgery went well until I received an alarming phone call from him the next day.

"Doc, I have a lot of pain going down my right arm into my hand, along with some numbness." He sounded worried. "It's hard for me to even move it. What should I do?" Mr. Thompson's livelihood depended on two functional arms. If he couldn't work because of pain, he could not pay the bills.

"Come by my office this afternoon and I will check you out." I had no idea why he would have pain down his arm. I thought the surgery went fine. I wasn't close to any of the major nerves in the area when I removed the lymph node. In my mind, there was no way I could have accidentally injured anything. There are patients I worry about for days because of something I might have come close to injuring during surgery, nervously awaiting the dreaded phone call. There are also bad outcomes from operations that do not surprise me when they manifest themselves several days later. During my career, I have caused some patients additional pain from complications. Most I have managed to correct. I would not have blamed a few if they had decided to sue me. Mr. Thompson's complaints took me by surprise. His operation was not one I was remotely concerned about.

I saw Mr. Thompson in my office and was terrified by what I found.

"Doc, it kills me to move my arm. I can't work like this." I continued to examine him as he spoke. "Did you injure a nerve or something?" I cringed. No surgeon likes to hear the words *nerve* and *injury* in the same sentence.

"To the best of my knowledge, no." I did not know what else to say. Once my examination was over, it was very clear to me that his complaints were consistent with some type of nerve injury. But for the life of me, I had no idea how this could have occurred during his surgery.

"Mr. Thompson, your symptoms are consistent with some type of partial nerve injury in the area where your lymph node was." I had to be honest with him. "I do not have an explanation as to how it could have happened. But I am responsible for it and sorry it has happened." He believed me because he felt I was honest and sincere. "I am going to have you see a neurologist and set up some physical therapy. Most of the time, symptoms like yours improve with time. Come back and see me in two weeks."

"Okay, Doc."

I have always tried to be honest with my patients when an operation does not end well. It is not easy to swallow professional pride, face the fear of legal retribution, and admit an imperfection. For years, the mantra of physicians was "Deny and defend!"

when it came to lawsuits, regardless of innocence or guilt. Most surgeons were thus indoctrinated because of the way the system punished their predecessors for mistakes. This way of thinking is still prevalent, despite the new attitudes encouraging surgeons to apologize and report their own errors. I believe most surgeons still have a difficult time admitting their mistakes. I also believe most surgeons still fear legal punishment for admitting errors. A 2008 study published by the *Archives of Internal Medicine* revealed that more than 90 percent of the physicians surveyed regarding medical errors stated (hypothetically) they would be likely to report a major error caused by their actions that resulted in disability or death. When queried about *real* major errors made in their practice, however, only 3.8 percent had actually reported the error. Despite the hypothetical inclination to admit to an error, only a handful of physicians have actually reported real ones.

Mr. Thompson left my office satisfied I was doing everything possible to help him. Despite knowing his arm pain would improve with time, I felt the legal sword of Damocles hanging over my head.

In my profession, lawsuits—justified or unjustified—are a fact of life. They are here to stay. Some doctors view every surgical patient who walks through the office door as a potential lawsuit. I am not that cynical. There are times when my evaluation of a patient for surgery incorporates the potential risk of a bad outcome along with the risk of getting sued. The reality of my work and the medical-legal climate I practice in forces me to think this way. As much as I would like, I cannot be perfect every time I step into the operating room. The medical literature bears this fact out. For example, if I perform 100 consecutive successful thyroid operations, the odds are very high that I will damage the nerve to the vocal cords in the 101st patient. This can result in permanent hoarseness and, in some situations, a lawsuit.

It doesn't matter if I had the best training in the world. It doesn't matter if I have the most experience in the world. Bad outcomes and unexpected deaths will continue to occur on my watch. They will continue to occur at your local hospital and at some of the most prestigious institutions in the country, as well.

If every surgeon practicing were "perfect," there would be no malpractice insurance to pay. There would be no malpractice lawyers to deal with. There would be no "medical malpractice economy"—an economy that exists because of the imperfections inherent in physicians, particularly surgeons. The malpractice economy has many components: malpractice insurance premiums, legal fees, settlement costs, and the cost of practicing defensive medicine in the office or hospital. This thriving economy is growing in many other ways, too. Even the most prestigious medical schools in the world have a stake in it. Now, many list courses on Liability Prevention for Physicians or A Physician's Guide to Surviving in Court in their brochures right under courses on updates in gastrointestinal cancer or surgery on the thyroid gland. It has gotten to the point where both courses are necessary for the working surgeon to stay competitive.

A recent study by Harvard researchers estimated that the medical liability system in this country (which includes all of the previously mentioned expenses) costs $55 billion annually.

To put this into perspective, this number alone is greater than the gross national product of many African and third-world countries.

Over the next three weeks, Mr. Thompson's arm pain improved dramatically with physical therapy and a little tender loving care. His lymph node biopsy turned out to be benign, and he was able to return to work full time. After he left my office for the last time, I turned to my partner Sam and vented. "I feel like I just dodged a major bullet."

"What do you mean?" Sam asked. I proceeded to fill him in on the story.

"Something is wrong with the system," I continued. "I feel more relieved about not getting sued than satisfied by helping my patient through his problem. How has it evolved to this? I don't see things getting any better."

"I know what you mean," Sam said. "How can the system ever change when there is a segment of the legal society perched waiting to punish us for our imperfections, for our misjudgments? I will never be at ease professionally without feeling the fear of a lawsuit whenever I have a bad outcome."

"Sam, ask any one of our colleagues and all will reluctantly tell you the same thing: Physicians are getting tired of fighting because not much is changing. There are no real national tort reforms. There are no disincentives to prevent unjust lawsuits from being filed. The vast majority of lawsuits filed end up getting dropped. Of those that go to court, the overwhelming majority are decided in favor of the physician. Despite this, I feel the lawyers are winning. Do you know, most nights when I watch television, I see commercials for malpractice lawyers. They're trolling for business. *Has your recent hip surgery gone bad? Was your breast cancer diagnosis delayed? Were you diagnosed with cerebral palsy at birth? Did your surgeon use this type of mesh during your hernia surgery?* How can I *not* practice defensive medicine out of fear when every night I see advertisements with malpractice lawyers looking to pay their kids' college tuition off my back? I can't escape this shit even in the confines of my own home."

"I know what you mean, Paul. I recently returned from a thyroid cancer conference with all the top experts in the world there. At the end of one of the lectures, a question was asked of the presenter: Why would she potentially overtreat a patient with early-stage thyroid cancer, despite the lack of credible support data? Her answer: *to keep the lawyers away.*"

"Sam, we are all being held hostage to a liability system that needs to change. The legal blanket suffocating our profession is getting heavier. Even today, surveys show that medical students graduating from medical school are going into specialties where they are less exposed to getting sued. I wish I had the answers for changing the practice climate of fear and eliminating frivolous lawsuits. All I know is I have a patient in the hospital with a bad complication from a recent surgery. I lie awake at night worrying about his recovery, worrying about making the right decisions. When I roll over in bed I also worry about getting sued."

Chapter 10

———————— /// ————————

Will Your Surgeon Be There?

"I can't wait to get out of this surgery business." I was exhausted. It was two in the morning with no end in sight to the work ahead. My hands were busy inside one of the worst abdomens I had ever been in, while my mind was struggling to stay awake. Several hours earlier, I had been called in by one of the gynecologists, Dr. Erin Jenkins, who was in the process of operating on her patient, Jane, for a gynecological emergency. Immediately after Dr. Jenkins opened Jane's abdomen, she realized she needed help from the general surgeon on call—me.

Jane's acutely diseased ovary was nestled deep in her pelvis, covered by a wad of immovable intestine. The problem was obvious: Everything in Jane's abdomen was encased with thick, leathery adhesions (scar tissue) from the bladder surgery she'd had as a child. Fingers of scar tissue held her intestines together like wads of gum stuck in someone's hair. It was nearly impossible to separate one segment from the next without tearing the intestine or making holes in its walls. Dr. Jenkins was not qualified to separate scar tissue like this (and accidentally cut holes in a patient's intestine). I was.

"Paul, you are too young to retire. You don't mean that, do you?" Erin was a well-liked, respected young ob/gyn surgeon in the community. Unfortunately, she had chosen to operate on a patient with an abdomen from hell. It was a hell we were descending into together while the rest of the world slept.

"On nights like this, yes, I do." My scissors slipped off some hard scar tissue and cut right through the wall of a loop of small intestine hiding behind it. "Shit. Nurse, three-oh Vicryl suture, please." I managed to pinch the hole off with my fingers before dark green liquid stool spilled out. The operation wasn't even close to completion and I was on enterotomy (hole) number three. There would be more. "Do you know that ten to fifteen percent of surgeons today, between ages fifty and sixty, are retiring early? A third of practicing surgeons today fall into this range. The average age of retirement is now under sixty." I sewed up the hole with the same fatigued, angry suture stroke that made me create it.

"If surgeons like you can't wait to get out, who is going to be left performing surgery? I read somewhere that ten thousand baby boomers are turning sixty-five every single day. People are living longer, and more will be requiring surgery as they age." Dr. Jenkins held the intestine steady while I closed the hole with a suture.

"That is the million-dollar question, Erin. Speaking of millions, who is going to be around to operate on the thirty to forty million *newly* insured people when they need a surgeon? Who is going to be showing up in the middle of the night to operate on a woman like this? Not me. I don't know where the future surgeons are going to come from. I don't know who they will be. I don't even know how confident or motivated they will be." I continued on the painstaking journey of cutting scar tissue, freeing up intestine, and intermittently making holes in Jane's intestine.

Since the mid-1990s, experts have predicted that there will be a significant shortage of surgeons in this country in the twenty-first century, a shortage knocking on the emergency room door right now. The numbers vary depending on which study you read. Yet in the end, all conclusions are the same: More surgeons will be needed. Over the next twenty years, the demand for surgical care will be robust for two reasons. One, because our booming age-sixty-five-and-older population will need it, and, two, because our increasingly insured population will want it. It boils down to supply and demand. The demand will be there, but the supply will not. Today, too many graduating medical students are *not* choosing careers in surgery—the training takes too many years, the on-call hours are long, and a career in surgery is not quality-of-life friendly. Newly minted doctors are looking for a nine-to-five job with minimal night calls, along with the potential to make big dollars. Close to half of medical school graduates today are women, and because most of them plan on starting families at some point, many decide not to travel down the long road of sacrifices it takes to become a surgeon, thus further depleting the potential ranks.

In addition to the unappealing quality-of-life issues, a career in surgery offers other reasons for medical school graduates to shy away from choosing to spend their working lives in an operating room. They see surgeons as "working too hard for too little money and too much risk" (both financial and physical). Other medical careers are far more appealing from a work/risk/reward perspective. Why not choose a medical specialty that affords the opportunity to make more money while working fewer hours and incurring less risk? Surgery is a high-risk profession. A recent *New England Journal of Medicine* study estimated 99 percent of general surgeons will have faced a malpractice lawsuit by age sixty-five.

Most surgery performed in this country is carried out at community hospitals by general surgeons, either in private practice or as employees of hospitals. As a general surgeon, I (like many of my colleagues) practice at a community hospital. As a surgeon in a private practice (I am not hospital-employed), I alone shoulder the legal risk every time I step into the operating room. Studies show that surgeons in private practice (whether solo or in a group) are more likely to get sued than surgeons working at well-known and named university hospitals. I believe this is because community surgeons are at greater legal risk simply because they do not have the intangible support attached to the reputations of the Harvards or Johns Hopkinses of the medical world.

A career in surgery can also be risky to your physical health. My job has an inherent hazard: My working tools are sharp needles and knives, both of which put me at risk when operating on patients with bloodborne infections, such as hepatitis B, hepatitis C, or H.I.V. A previous survey of surgeons in training revealed that 99 percent of them experienced an average of eight accidental needlesticks during their five years of training. Of those who reported the incidents, 53 percent involved a needlestick contaminated by patients who were at high risk for (or were *known* to have) hepatitis B or C or H.I.V. During his last month of training, my chief resident accidentally stuck himself with a needle while operating on a patient with H.I.V. Needless to say, he was a mental basket case for days and had to take powerful medicine for weeks afterward. He ended up being fine (physically), but the trauma to his psyche took some work to heal. Today, graduating medical students are factoring in all of these risks when deciding on a specialty, and more and more that means not choosing a career in surgery.

///

"Paul, what do you think about the surgeons coming out of training today? Obviously there will not be enough of them. But will the ones coming out of training even be able to handle the long hours, the older, more complicated patients, and the high-pressure situations?" Dr. Jenkins was trying to help me move along by keeping the conversation going. She was exhausted as well.

"Yes, Erin, these are more million-dollar questions, especially since the eighty-hour workweek is here to stay." Since 2003, new guidelines for surgical residents require that they work *no more than twenty-four hours straight* (sixteen hours straight for interns), and eighty hours total a week. The rules were instituted to cut down on mistakes caused by fatigue, to encourage more learning, and to improve quality of life. I laughed as I cut another hole in Jane's intestine.

"Why are you laughing, Paul?" Dr. Jenkins was puzzled. I laughed because it took less energy than crying.

"Erin, I trained in a totally different era and I am not that old. There was never a limit on the number of hours I could work. There was no clock to punch. On the contrary, it was a sign of strength to stay up as long as possible. Sure, after about a hundred hours, everything was a blur, but it was a character-building blur. It may not have been good for my patients *then*, but it is good for them now. I would have lived at the hospital around the clock just to take advantage of the opportunity to get into the operating room. For me, it was an obsession. Nothing else mattered. Sleeping, eating, even going to the bathroom were luxuries. Most nights I was lucky to do two out of the three." I was finally making some progress cutting through the scar tissue. "Forget about reading and learning from books. I learned on the job and at all hours. When I did get the chance to read, the sound of the open book hitting the floor usually woke me up."

"But, Paul, I can understand their concerns, wanting to cut down on the mistakes residents make. Patient safety must come first. Studies have shown that after working twenty-four hours straight, fatigue does lead to mistakes."

"I don't need a study to tell me that. Mistakes happen when you are wide awake and when you're tired. I made my share during training. It didn't matter whether I was tired or not. But the process forces you to deal with fatigue, forces you to dig deep and concentrate in the face of unrelenting adversity. It was preparing us for the real world of surgery. It was preparing me for nights like tonight. Patients don't stop needing surgery after eight P.M., you know." It was now three in the morning. My eyes were hurting.

"Paul, wouldn't you want someone fresh, alert operating on you?" Dr. Jenkins was playing devil's advocate.

"No. I want someone who knows what the hell they are doing . . ." It was her turn to laugh. "What about me, as a surgeon in private practice? I now have been up for twenty-two hours and have another eight hours of elective operations in front of me. I would love to be home right now in bed. I don't have a choice as a practicing surgeon. It's not realistic behavior, though, if I'm going to make a living or build a practice. The eighty-hour-workweek rule applies only to residents. They can go home because someone will step in to take their place. Wait until they get out into my world! I had no choice but to come in and help you. I accept that I am not my mental best when operating tired. I also realize I have the experience to do it, if forced to. I know studies have suggested that less than six hours of sleep increases a surgeon's complication rate the next day. What choice do I have? All I can do is suck it up, down some coffee, and do the best I can." I paused. "Erin, you do know what the real issue surrounding the eighty-hour workweek is, don't you?"

"No, Paul. What is it?" She really did not know.

"The real issue focuses light on the competency of surgeons coming out of training today. Are their reduced work hours limiting their operative experience enough to affect their competency? That is the big elephant in the room." I continued to methodically massage scar tissue with my fingers, thinning it out, cutting it, and then separating the involved intestine. Massage, cut, and separate. My life was condensed to three simple physical movements at three in the morning.

"Has that been proven to be an issue?" Dr. Jenkins asked.

"Depends whom you ask." I was not kidding. "Right now, published studies have not shown an appreciable decrease in operative experience (the number of cases) for finishing surgical residents, or enough to raise a flag about competency. I think the jury is still out because it is going to take time to show itself. We already have plenty of data for some major operations, showing that a surgeon's volume experience is inversely proportional to his or her operative mortality rates. If I am not doing enough pancreatic resections, heart bypasses, aneurysm repairs, esophageal resections, or lung resections, my patients will die at a higher rate." Dr. Jenkins kept listening. "I did read something interesting last week."

"What was it?" she asked.

"I came across a study stating that eighty percent of graduating surgical chief residents are going on to more training, or fellowships, before going out into the real world to practice."

"What does that tell you?" she asked.

"It *could* tell me that the future surgeons who will be operating on you and me when we turn sixty-five do not feel confident enough, despite what their experience is on paper, to start practicing independently. It could also tell me that our future surgeons want to be 'specialist surgeons,' concentrating on a limited number of specific operations. Like the data proves, the more operations of a specific type I perform, the better I get at them. Surgeons today want to concentrate on operating on one body part, repair one organ, or replace one joint. This approach is efficient, less stressful, and very predictable. The good news is you only have to worry about one body part while someone else worries about the rest of the patient."

"What is the bad news?" Dr. Jenkins asked.

"You only worry about one body part while someone else worries about the rest of the patient." I wasn't kidding.

"Why is that bad news?" She was puzzled.

"It limits what type of operations you will want to get involved with or feel confident doing. If or when you are forced to stray beyond your comfort zone in the operating room, outcomes may not be perfect. Too many specialists also means higher costs.

"Overall, surgical specialists, such as oncologic surgeons and colorectal surgeons, are paid more money and can argue for being on call less because they are specialists and only deal with problems in their area of expertise, which are generally not going to present as emergencies that need a surgeon in the middle of the night." I paused. "If I were in that group, I would be in bed right now."

"I'm sorry." Dr. Jenkins felt bad, but she'd had no choice other than to call me in when she did. She knew she needed help, for the good of the patient. As a general surgeon, I make a living cutting scar tissue and fondling intestine inside the abdomen.

I am not considered a specialist surgeon. I am considered a jack-of-all-trades surgeon. I pay the bills by draining pus, removing lumps, cutting scar tissue, taking out gallbladders, operating on trauma, repairing hernias, removing cancerous colons, performing appendectomies, and dealing with whatever else needs surgical attention in the emergency room.

Another hour had passed. We both were still standing, varicose veins and all. Our hands kept working. There was no way to hurry the process of freeing up this woman's intestine. The faster I tried to go, the more holes I would come close to making. Dr. Jenkins and I were cellmates, prisoners to this woman's angry, merciless, scarred abdomen. There was little chance of making parole before the sun came up.

"Erin, ask any surgeon today if he or she would go into surgery again, if given the opportunity. Many will give you the same answer. 'No! I should have gone to business school.' " I looked up at the clock. A chill came over me. "You have children, don't you?"

"Yes, why do you ask?" She looked up at my eyes.

"Would you encourage your children to go into medicine or surgery today?"

"Paul, I would have to think about that." She smiled beneath her mask.

"What is there to think about? Many surgeons, after ten years of practice, secretly can't wait to get out of the business they worked so hard to get into." It's ironic. I was willing to sacrifice most of my twenties and thirties to school and training, waiting for the day when I could put up my own shingle. I could feel the weight of the early-morning hour pressuring my eyeballs. I had to keep talking. My hands were moving by themselves, on auto-pilot. My eyes were focused in front of me, but I wasn't clearly seeing where I was pointing my scissors.

"Would you retire next week if you could?" Erin already knew the answer to her question.

"Of course I would. I would if I had the money in the bank to live the lifestyle I wanted to. You know that many of us will continue to work like dogs for years, though. We sacrifice our personal lives, our health, putting money away, hoping our investments grow so we can afford to retire early."

"Paul, don't you enjoy operating?" Erin asked.

"Not at four in the morning." Erin laughed. "Of course, truthfully, that is why I went into surgery—I enjoy it. Lately though, some days I do, some days I don't. When operations go well, the feeling of satisfaction is a unique high that no recreational drug can do justice to. When they don't, no narcotic in the world can ease the emotional pain. When I have good news to give a patient about an optimistic survival rate after his or her cancer was removed, I relish my job. When I open up a thirty-nine-year-old man and find cancer everywhere, I fear it." I managed to abruptly stop my scissors, right before nearly cutting another hole in yet another piece of intestine.

"Why do you think so many surgeons are retiring early?" Erin asked.

"Where do you want me to start?" I briefly stepped back from the table, shook the cobwebs from my head. I had several elective operations starting in three and a half hours and I needed to stay awake. There wasn't going to be any time for sleep. It was going to be a long day. I wanted to get through it without hurting anyone.

"Erin, the list is long. It starts with burnout from working longer hours, operating in the middle of the night, taking care of complicated older, sicker patients. Some days I have to catch myself for thinking every diseased gallbladder or cancerous colon gets me one more operation closer to retirement." I paused.

"Do you really think that?" Erin asked.

"Yes, when burnout comes calling. There are some days I'm just too mentally tired to see another cancer or sick appendix." I was being honest.

"What are some of the other reasons?" she asked.

"Start with rising malpractice insurance rates, fatigue from living under the threat of potential lawsuits, decreasing reimbursements, increased government regulation, and losing whatever autonomy I have left." I continued to methodically cut through scar tissue, untwisting intestine while thinking about breakfast. There is something erotic about eating two eggs over easy, sausage, home fries, and toast after staying up all night.

The American College of Surgeons Committee on Physician Competency and Health surveyed close to eight thousand surgeons about their job satisfaction and mental state. The results revealed that 40 percent of those who answered the survey met the criteria for "burnout." The publishers of the study attributed this burnout to increased working hours, being on call, and the job's effect on home life. In addition, some studies have suggested burnout to be predictive of future mistakes made by surgeons.

It is intuitive, really: Burned-out surgeons have a greater potential to make more mistakes in the operating room.

The survey also uncovered that 30 percent of those who responded screened positive for depression. This was made worse by working more than eighty hours per week. Along with this information, the survey discovered a higher rate of thoughts of suicide in surgeons over age forty-five—1.5 to 3 times that of the general population. Of those who reported suicidal thoughts, two-thirds were reluctant to seek help for fear of reprisals to their practice or medical license.

"Erin, having to come and operate in the middle of the night gets old quickly. I didn't pay much attention to it early in my practice and could shake it off easily. Now it takes me several days to recover from a night like this, several days of feeling like shit. It is several days of being no use to anyone, including my wife. The problem is I can't afford to lose several days of business." I could sense I was getting close to uncovering Jane's ovaries because I was running out of intestine to free up. "Erin, don't you get tired of coming in late at night?" Dr. Jenkins was an ob/gyn and I suspected her hours to be longer than mine.

"Of course I do. It sucks having to drag yourself out of a nice warm bed. Yet it's part of the job, part of what I signed up for." She was right.

"Erin"—I was probing—"what do you think you and I will get paid for this operation? After seven hours in this woman's abdomen, what do you think Medicare would pay us?"

"I have no idea," she responded.

"I don't want to know. I suspect it will be less than what my plumber makes for just stepping into my house. What about Medicaid?" I pushed.

"Again, I have no idea." She was honest.

"Erin, it's close to zero. I must be honest with you; I am getting tired of operating and taking on all the risks for close to zero. I do it because my training, my oath, obligates me to do it." I paused. "There will come a point when I, and many of my colleagues, will not be able to afford to operate on Medicare and Medicaid patients. Whatever I get for being here seven hours, it will not be enough for the time, stress, and fatigue I have invested, and will continue to invest, in this woman. If she doesn't do well, we are also at risk. Erin, what do you pay in malpractice premiums?"

Erin paused. "It is over six figures."

"I am not surprised. Frankly, I don't know how you do it. My premiums rise despite having a clean record. I am fed up with having to pay more money to these insurance companies every year. I am also tired of living under the cloud of a malpractice lawsuit every time I have a bad outcome. Erin, I heard that one of your colleagues, several years ago, was taking care of a high-risk pregnancy in a woman with no insurance." She did not say a thing. "He did the best he could, given the situation. I guess there was a bad outcome with the baby and the woman turned around and sued him. Shit like this wears on you. You bust your balls with good intentions and then you have to deal with this." There wasn't much small intestine left to separate. I was almost at the end, at the connection to the large intestine. I managed to push all of what I had freed up out of the pelvis.

"Finally, six hours later and there they are. That is the best thing I have seen all month." Jane's ovaries were staring us in the face. One was very hemorrhagic (bleeding) and had to be removed. It was my turn now to help Erin do what she had been waiting seven hours to do: remove an ovary.

I stayed an extra twenty minutes to help Dr. Jenkins take out the woman's ovary. Once it was out, my work was done. "Erin, I'm out of here." I looked at the clock. It was six forty-five in the morning. I had forty-five minutes to shower, shave, and have breakfast before starting my "scheduled" operations. After a quick hot shower, I made the mistake of sitting down in a chair, resting my head back, and allowing my eyelids to succumb to gravity. *I can't do this . . . need to get up. I have another six hours of operating ahead and need to wake up. These patients have waited weeks for their surgery. I cannot let them down.* I slapped my face a few times. *Should I tell my first patient I have been up all night? Should I give her the option of canceling her surgery?* So much for my eighty-hour workweek.

With the supply of surgeons decreasing because fewer medical school graduates are going into surgery and more surgeons are retiring early, who will be left? Who is going to come in the middle of the night to perform emergency surgery and continue to care for you afterward?

After inhaling my two eggs, sausage, home fries, and toast over two cups of coffee, I quickly ran up to the floor to see a consult. I had been paged to see a forty-five-year-old woman with abdominal pain and gallstones. She was admitted through the emergency room last night under one of the hospitalists. Her family physician gave up his admitting privileges last year and no longer admitted patients to the hospital. He, like many of his colleagues, made a business/lifestyle decision to concentrate on an office practice. With more medical doctors relinquishing their admitting privileges to local hospitals, who is left to care for patients? Today, community hospitals employ "hospitalists" to care for admitted patients. Hospitalists are qualified internal medicine physicians who work in shifts, covering admitted hospital patients twenty-four hours a day. They are your personal doctors while you are being cared for in the hospital. They are the ones making the decisions about your care during their shifts. Many are highly qualified physicians, although they often remain nameless (and faceless) to the patients they care for. But hospitalists do not know anything about you until you get admitted. They get paid for taking care of your acute illnesses *inside* the hospital, leaving it up to your family doctor to see you for follow-up care. One of the goals of all hospitalists is to reduce your stay in the hospital and get you on your way.

Despite the break in continuity of care, hospitalists are necessary and have become the standard of medical care today. They are one answer to the growing shortage of primary care physicians in this country. Yet with hospitalists, the continuity of care offered by a long-standing family doctor is broken. Each day in the hospital, you see a different face, a different hospitalist who was given a report on your condition by the preceding hospitalist. As a patient, you get "handed off" to the next hospitalist. With handoffs comes the potential for breakdowns in communication. With breakdowns in communication comes the potential for medical errors.

/ / /

As I sat there, looking through the woman's chart, I did not recognize the hospitalist physician's name on her chart. *Must be a new group hired by the hospital. I can never keep track of these guys.* As I looked at her lab tests, I thought, *Will this happen to surgery in the future?* It is possible. Will private practice surgeons be replaced by surgeon hospitalists? This is also possible. Will a surgeon hospitalist, a part-time hired gun employed by the hospital to fill a need, operate on you in the middle of the night and then leave by sunup? Most likely. What will you know about his or her credentials or experience? Nothing. Only the hospital will know. Will this surgeon-hospitalist have a vested interest in you as a person or view you as a job: a diseased gallbladder, a hot appendix, or an incarcerated hernia? Will he or she hand off your care to the next surgeon hospitalist the following morning like a loaf of bread? Probably.

After I finished examining the patient, it was obvious that her symptoms were caused by gallstones. She needed to have her gallbladder removed. It was very straightforward. The problem was that I did not have the time that day, or the energy, to do it.

"Doctor, when do you think you can do her surgery?" the patient's nurse wanted to know.

"When?" I was exhausted. "What about *if*?" I said as I began to walk away. Despite being up all night, I could not turn down

a perfectly healthy patient with a diseased gallbladder ripe for plucking. I had no choice but to add her on the schedule today. Tomorrow's schedule was even worse. *There is no way I am going to keep this pace up the next twenty years.* I just can't see myself operating into my late sixties or early seventies unless I am dirt broke, get divorced, or develop a gambling problem. First, I know that my stamina and tolerance for being woken up in the middle of the night or operating long hours will not last. Second, my surgical skills will probably not be there, at least not the way I would like them to be. I already see the subtle signs. My eyesight (even though fine with glasses) is not what it was ten years ago. My hand steadiness is aging just like the rest of my body. Cognitively, I am still sharp but my desire to learn "new techniques" is in desperate need of some Viagra. I don't know how some of my older colleagues stay sharp and operate with all the vigor they displayed right out of training. Many, like my senior partner, are from a different generation and represent a different breed of surgeon from the ones now being produced. I greatly admire their lifelong dedication to patients and their ability to survive so long. (I know I come close to the former but will never equal the latter.) I am grateful they are still around because they may be the only ones left.

The aging surgeon population is a creeping problem in this country, one that may present unique challenges ahead. Some surgeons' physical and mental skills age better than others. The lifestyle of a surgeon is physically and emotionally demanding, especially when you factor in being on call. Many older surgeons voluntarily decide, once they reach a certain age, to no longer take emergency calls wherever they practice. This is their right from a hospital-privilege point of view and from a tradition point of view. As the surgeon population ages, more will opt out of emergency calls, leaving them to the younger "guns" to make up the slack. Unfortunately, there may not be enough younger surgeons to step up and be counted.

"Doctor, you ordered the wrong antibiotic if she is going to the operating room." I had one foot in the elevator when the nurse shouted down the corridor at me. She was correct. "The one you ordered is not part of the S.C.I.P. protocol. You must order the antibiotic stated in the hospital S.C.I.P. protocol or the hospital will get dinged."

"Yes, how could I forget? I must abide by the S.C.I.P. protocol or the hospital will not get paid." I was being sarcastic. I knew all about the S.C.I.P. protocol and its growing influence on physician behavior and hospital reimbursements.

"Doctor, do you want to order prophylaxis to prevent deep vein clots before her surgery as per the S.C.I.P. protocol?" she asked again.

"Do I have to?" I continued the sarcasm. The patient's nurse was not happy. "No, not yet. I will order the medication after the operation." I closed the elevator door behind me.

"Don't forget to document it in the chart. J.C.A.H.O. will be here next week." J.C.A.H.O. (pronounced "jay-co") stands for the Joint Commission (formerly called the Joint Commission on Accreditation of Healthcare Organizations, now simply T.J.C.). Her voice was following me down to the ground floor. How could I forget? This is the mother of all hospital licensing bodies, with absolute authority. Technically, it is a private, nonprofit organization, but the federal government uses its seal of approval as gospel. Every three years, hospitals have to undergo a Joint Commission inspection in order to qualify for federal Medicaid and Medicare dollars. In today's competitive healthcare business, the blessing of a T.J.C. inspection is a necessity. Hospitals jump through enormous hoops to pass and receive their coveted seal of approval. The process is so intense, with so much at stake, hospital administrators have been fired over failed Joint Commission inspections.

The Joint Commission inspects *everything*—the completeness of a patient's chart, documentation of a physician's orders, the legibility of a physician's signature, the dirt on the walls of a patient's room. T.J.C. inspectors bring their federally blessed guidelines and recommendations into every corner of every hospital, including my world—the operating room. These guidelines are shaping the way I practice surgery today.

The Surgical Care Improvement Project (S.C.I.P.) best-practices initiative is a national alliance of organizations brought together to improve the safety of the surgical patient. The project was initiated in 2003 by the Centers for Medicare & Medicaid Services (C.M.S., part of the U.S. Department of Health and Human Services) and the Centers for Disease Control and Prevention (C.D.C.). This was also when the increase in federal regulations over the way physicians practice (including the eighty-hour workweek) all started. As a body, the organizations involved under S.C.I.P. produced guidelines, checklists, and protocols based on medical evidence aimed at reducing the incidence of complications and death in the surgical patient. Some of the guidelines mandate the use of antibiotics before and after surgery, the use of medicine to decrease the risk of a heart attack during surgery and to reduce the incidence of blood clots to the leg and lung (pulmonary embolus). Checklists used inside the operating room to reduce the incidence of errors have also been mandated by S.C.I.P. for all hospitals. All hospitals (and their staff physicians) have been mandated to follow S.C.I.P. guidelines in the name of patient safety and, of course, in the name of getting paid.

After getting off the elevator, I made my way to the preoperative area to say hello to my first elective surgery patient. "Hello, Mrs. Fielding. I need to mark the left side of your neck, corresponding to the left thyroid gland I am going to remove." This was T.J.C. requirement number one, an attempt to prevent wrong-site surgery. I proceeded to place a *yes* with a marker on the left side of her neck. She had a "suspicious thyroid nodule on biopsy." It needed to be removed. I next had to verify, sign, date, and time my history and physical (H&P) form in her chart (T.J.C. requirement number two).

"Dr. Ruggieri, did you get a good night's sleep last night?" she asked.

"No, not really, Mrs. Fielding. But you will be fine." Her husband looked at me. I had to be honest with her.

"I trust you," she said.

"Okay, let's go. I will meet you in the operating room." After I left, the nurses went down their checklists, making sure all the paperwork was in order.

Once inside the operating room, a "time out" was done with the participation of Mrs. Fielding while she was awake, lying on her stretcher. A time out is done to verify verbally who the patient is, who the surgeon is, and what the procedure is going to be, as well as what side the surgery is going to be on (T.J.C. requirement number three). I comply with it because I have no choice. At the end, the nurses, the anesthesiologist, and the surgeon have to verify together with the words "I agree." The exercise is supposed to promote the "team" concept of surgery, getting everyone involved, with the hope of reducing errors inside the operating room. Studies have shown that a time out in the operating room *does* reduce the number of errors. Along with the time out, the team approach to surgery is here to stay.

I have reluctantly embraced the team concept for several reasons, the main one being I have no choice. Deep down, my raw instincts as a surgeon do not embrace being on a team. My surgeon heritage is rich with individuals who are independent, strong-willed, and borderline psychotic; hate being questioned; and rule as masters of their domains. These are hardly characteristics of team players, especially if the team is viewed as inferior. I went into surgery so I could rely on my own instincts and skills, not the team's. As a surgeon, I consider myself a loner. If I wanted to be on a team, I would have gone into hospital administration. I do not look kindly into putting my patient's life in the hands of "a team." When it is two in the morning and the only thing standing between a patient with a ruptured spleen and death is my skills, there is no time to be a member of a team. When I have a bad outcome and expose myself to legal action, is there a team to share the liability? No. I alone am, and want to be, the one in control. The operating room is my kingdom, my workplace. I want to make the rules. I resent anyone telling me what I need to be doing. The older generation of surgeons, in which I count myself, is having a difficult time being part of a team. It is just not in our nature.

"That time out we just did seemed a little long. Was more added to it?" I asked.

"Yes, more verification questions were added by J.C.A.H.O.," a nurse volunteered. I should have known. Once Mrs. Fielding was asleep, her neck was draped off. Before I could grab the knife, another time out had to be done verifying the same information we had just verified five minutes ago (T.J.C. requirement number four).

"Everyone agree?" the lead nurse asked.

"What has changed from five minutes ago?" I love saying this. "Why do we need to repeat this?" It was hospital policy.

Mrs. Fielding's operation went well. At the end of her surgery, however, the scrub nurse had an incorrect needle count. Incorrect needle counts can happen. In abdominal surgery, needles can get lost inside the abdomen. In thyroid surgery, however, using a four-inch incision, the chance of a needle getting lost is virtually zero.

"Hold it. Dr. Ruggieri, we need to get an x-ray to see if the needle is in the patient's neck before we wake her up." I could feel a wave of fatigue coming on.

"Listen, I can tell you there is no needle in that woman's neck. I can tell you this because I was the one using all the needles.

You know it and I know it." I was getting testy. "What are the chances of me losing a needle in a four-inch incision? Forget the x-ray. I will take responsibility for this. It is a waste of time and money."

"I am sorry, Dr. Ruggieri, we have to get an x-ray. It is hospital policy. It doesn't matter what you think. You have no choice." She was right and I was tired. "Plus, if I don't order an x-ray, I will get in trouble." She was right again.

"Fine, get the x-ray, keep the patient under anesthesia for another twenty minutes for no good reason. Go ahead, expose her to needless radiation. Go ahead, throw away some more health-care dollars." I threw my hands up in the air. "I only work here. My opinion doesn't matter anyway." With that, I left the room, knowing full well the x-ray was not going to show a missing needle. It didn't. The patient was charged with the cost of an extra twenty minutes of anesthesia and an x-ray. The original needle count was incorrect. Everyone knew it, yet the x-ray had to be done.

Today, everything in healthcare is becoming standardized: office practices, tests ordered, the treatment of disease. Diagnostic and treatment decisions are being taken out of a physician's hands by mandated hospital policies handed down by the national governing bodies that control the reimbursement checkbooks (such as C.M.S.). Because of these policies, physician behavior and decision making is, begrudgingly, changing. It is changing because hospitals (and physicians) are being forced to show 100 percent compliance or they will not get paid. The room for independent thinking by seasoned physicians (especially surgeons) is shrinking. The days when a surgeon's word in regard to his or her patient's care was gospel are disappearing with each new policy and regulation. I have been accustomed to dictating the terms of my profession and controlling the workplace when it involved my patients. Today, the control I once had is diminishing. The art of practicing medicine and surgery is slowly losing its creativity. It seems that more and more of what I do is being regulated and scrutinized by state or federal organizations thousands of miles away.

The Joint Commission, S.C.I.P., and C.M.S. are all organizations born out of the genuine need and desire to reduce medical errors, improve patient care, and reduce costs. These regulations have already invaded every aspect of my office practice (from billing to patient care), from the minute a patient walks in to the day I get paid. Regulations are also causing surgeons to frequently look over their shoulder in the operating room to see who is watching. In the future, I believe surgeons will be forced to prove their competency far beyond what is called for today. Surgeons don't like to be forced to do anything, especially when it comes to providing proof of their own skills. The future surgeons of America will eventually have to present a report card on competency for every operation they want to perform. Personally, I believe this would be beneficial, and I would embrace further regulation toward this goal. However, many competent surgeons who trained in a different era, an era when they made the rules and no one questioned their word, may have a difficult time with this.

I believe the day will come, unfortunately, when regulatory policies and protocols are going to dictate to me whom to operate on, where to cut, how long my operation should take, what instruments to use, and how much time I am allowed to spend on each operation. Someday, there will come a time when a regulatory entity will figuratively take the scalpel blade right out of my hand. When that day arrives, there will be no more surgeons left to do the cutting.

Bibliography

Asch, D. A., and R. H. Parker. "The Libby Zion Case." *New England Journal of Medicine* 318 (1988): 771–75.

Bishop, T. F., et al. "Physicians' Views on Defensive Medicine: A National Survey." *Archives of Internal Medicine* 170 (2010): 1081–83.

Carter, P. L. "Remembering Dr. Jim Gillespie." *American Journal of Surgery* 201 (2011): 561–64.

DesRoches, C. "Physicians' Perceptions, Preparedness for Reporting, and Experiences Related to Impaired and Incompetent Colleagues." *JAMA* 3409 (2010): 187–93.

Gawande, A. A., et al. "Analysis of Errors Reported by Surgeons at Three Teaching Hospitals." *Surgery* 133 (2003): 614–21.

Jena, A. B., et al. "Malpractice Risk According to Physician Specialty." *New England Journal of Medicine* 365 (2011): 629–36.

Kaldjian, L. C., et al. "Reporting Medical Errors to Improve Patient Safety." *Archives of Internal Medicine* 168 (2010): 40–45.

Kohn, L. T., J. M. Corrigan, and M. S. Donaldson, eds. *To Err Is Human.* Washington, D.C.: National Academy Press, 1999.

Makary, M. "Needle Stick Injuries." *New England Journal of Medicine* 356 (2007): 2693–99.

Mello, M., et al. "National Costs of the Medical Liability System." *Health Affairs* 29 (September 2010): 1569–77.

Rothschild, J. M., et al. "Risk of Complications by Attending Physicians after Performing Nighttime Procedures." *JAMA* 302 (2009): 1565–72.

Shanafelt, T. D., et al. "Burnout and Career Satisfaction among American Surgeons." *Annals of Surgery* 250 (2009): 463–71.

———. "Burnout and Medical Errors among American Surgeons." *Annals of Surgery* 251 (2010): 995–1000.

———. "Suicidal Ideation among American Surgeons." *Annals of Surgery* 146 (2011): 54–62.

Shoianna, K. G. "Changes in Rates of Autopsy-Detected Diagnostic Errors over Time." *JAMA* 289 (2003): 2849–56.

Studdert, D. M., et al. "Defensive Medicine among High-Risk Specialist Physicians in a Volatile Malpractice Environment." *JAMA* 293 (2005): 2609–17.

Sullivan, M. "DataWatch." *American College of Surgeons Surgery News* 7 (2011): 1–4.

Walker, E. "Replacement Rates Vary for Aging Surgeon Population." *American College of Surgeons Surgery News* 1 (2011): 17–19.